AICOG 2023 Workshop Manual

Solutions for the Subfertile Couple

A Clinician's Handbook

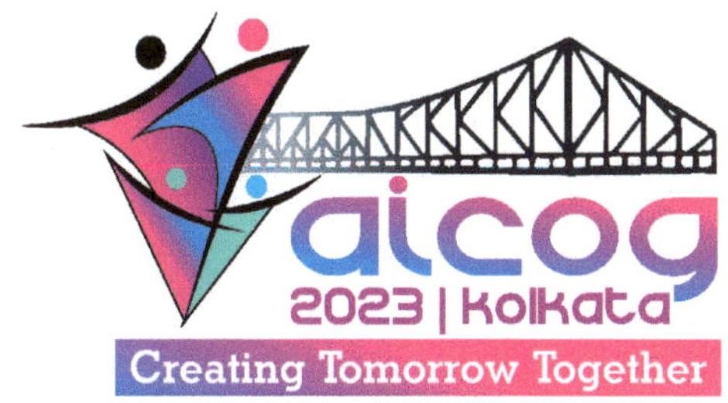

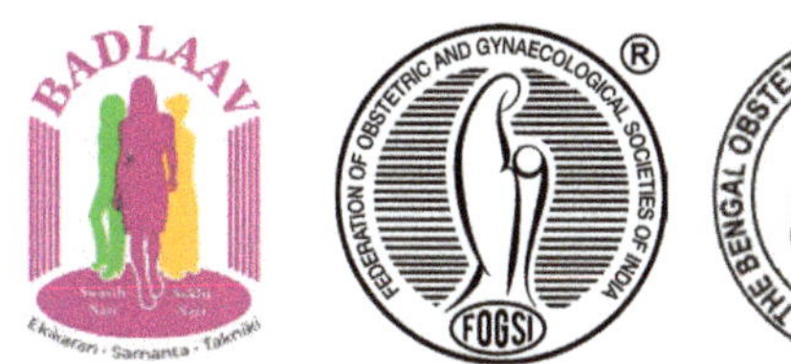

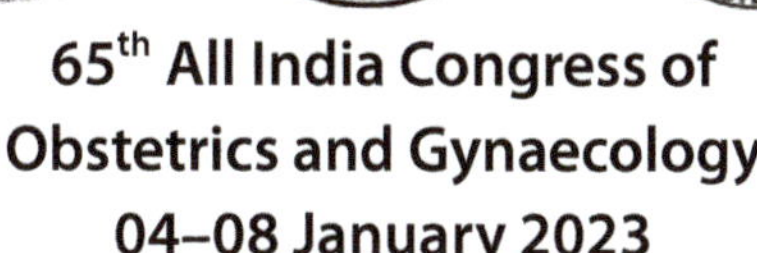

65th All India Congress of
Obstetrics and Gynaecology
04–08 January 2023

AICOG 2023 Workshop Manual

Solutions for the Subfertile Couple

A Clinician's Handbook

Series Editors

Bhaskar Pal
Basab Mukherjee
Dibyendu Banerjee
Kusagradhi Ghosh

Volume Editors

Chaitali Datta Ray
Kausiki Ray Sarkar
Sudip Basu
Sujoy Dasgupta

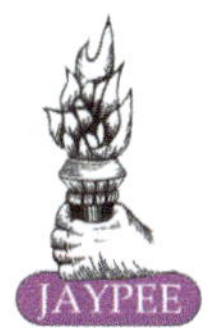

JAYPEE BROTHERS MEDICAL PUBLISHERS
The Health Sciences Publisher
New Delhi | London

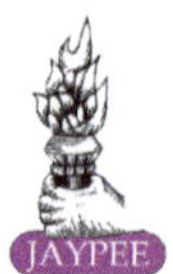 **Jaypee Brothers Medical Publishers (P) Ltd**

Headquarters

Jaypee Brothers Medical Publishers (P) Ltd
EMCA House, 23/23-B
Ansari Road, Daryaganj
New Delhi 110 002, India
Landline: +91-11-23272143, +91-11-23272703
+91-11-23282021, +91-11-23245672
Email: jaypee@jaypeebrothers.com

Corporate Office

Jaypee Brothers Medical Publishers (P) Ltd
4838/24, Ansari Road, Daryaganj
New Delhi 110 002, India
Phone: +91-11-43574357
Fax: +91-11-43574314
Email: jaypee@jaypeebrothers.com

Overseas Office

JP Medical Ltd
83 Victoria Street, London
SW1H 0HW (UK)
Phone: +44 20 3170 8910
Fax: +44 (0)20 3008 6180
Email: info@jpmedpub.com

Website: www.jaypeebrothers.com
Website: www.jaypeedigital.com

AICOG 2023 Workshop Manual: Solutions for the Subfertile Couple— A Clinician's Handbook

First Edition: 2023

ISBN: 978-93-5696-124-1

Contributors

Ameet Patki MD DNB FICOG FCPS FRCOG (UK)
Medical Director
IKAN Fertility Associates
Mumbai, Maharashtra, India
Former Hon Associate Professor
KJ Somaiya Medical College and Hospital
Country Representative
President Elect, ISAR
Past Chair, West Zone AICC RCOG
Past President, Mumbai Obstetrics and
Gynaecological Society

Arnav Pai MD
Mumbai, Maharashtra, India

Asha Baxi MBBS FICOG FRCOG MS
Consultant Obstetrician,
Gynecologist and Infertility Specialist
Disha Fertility Centre
Indore, Madhya Pradesh, India

Chaitali Datta Ray MD FICOG
Professor
Department of Obstetrics and
Gynecology
Institute of Postgraduate Medical
Education and Research
Kolkata, West Bengal, India
Member, State Appropriate Authority
West Bengal (ART & Surrogacy Act)
Managing Committee Member and
Quiz Coordinator, Bengal Obstetric and
Gynecological Society
UNICEF Consultant on
"Transforming of Labor Rooms"
Trainer of LAQSHYA, NSSK, KMC, MAA
and PPIUCD
Invited Expert for Evaluation of
Scholars, IIT Kharagpur

Fessy Louis MBBS DGO DNB MNAM
Senior Consultant and Additional
Professor
Department of Reproductive
Medicine and Surgery
Amrita Fertility Centre
Amrita Institute of Medical Sciences
Kochi, Kerala, India

Geetendra Sharma MD (Obs & Gyne)
LLB (Gold Medalist)
Obstetrician and Gynecologist and
Medicolegal Practitioner
Ahmedabad, Gujarat, India
Vice President, FOGSI (2022–23)

Hrishikesh D Pai MD FRCOG FCPS
FICOG MSc (USA)
Gynecologist and Head of IVF Unit
Lilavati Hospital
Mumbai, Maharashtra, India
Consultant Gynecologist
Fortis Bloom IVF Centers at Fortis La
Femme and Fortis Memorial Hospital
Gurugram, Haryana, India

Jaideep Malhotra MD FICMCH FICOG
FRCOG FRCPI FMAS
Managing Director
ART Rainbow IVF and MNMH (P) Ltd
Ujala Cygnus Rainbow Hospital
Agra, Uttar Pradesh, India
President, SAFOM/ISPAT

Jyotsana Singh MS Fellowship in
Reproductive Medicine
Consultant
Bloom IVF Centre
Mumbai, Maharashtra, India

Kalpana Udupa MD (Obs & Gyne)
Senior Resident
Department of Obstetrics and
Gynecology
Lakhimpur Medical College
and Hospital
Lakhimpur, Assam, India

Kausiki Ray Sarkar DNB DGO
Fellowship in Rep Endocrinology and Infertility
(ISRAEL)
In-charge
Fertility Unit
AMRI Medical Centre
Kolkata, West Bengal, India

Khyati Pandya MBBS DGO
Clinical Fellow
IKAN Fertility Associates
Mumbai, Maharashtra, India

Manisha T Kundnani MD FNB FNUS
Founder Director and Chief Fertility
Specialist
Fertility Square
Mumbai, Maharashtra, India
Joint Secretary, FOGSI 2022–23

Nandita Palshetkar MD FCPS FICOG
FRCOG (UK)
Medical Director and Infertility
Specialist
Bloom IVF
Fortis LaFemme Hospital
New Delhi, India

Pranay Phukan MD FICOG
Associate Professor
Assam Medical College and Hospital
Dibrugarh, Assam, India

Rajeev Agarwal MD (Obs & Gyne)
Director
Renew Healthcare
Kolkata, West Bengal, India

Rishma Dhillon Pai MD FRCOG DNB
FCPS DGO FICOG
Consultant Gynecologist
Lilavati, Jaslok and Hinduja Hospitals
Mumbai, Maharashtra, India
Treasurer, International Federation of
Fertility Societies IFFS
Former President, FOGSI, ISAR, IAGE,
MOGS

Rohan Palshetkar MBBS MS
Infertility Specialist
Babies and US Fertility IVF Centre
Mumbai, Maharashtra, India

Shiuli Mukherjee MBBS MS FNB
Director
Mukherjee Fertility Centre
Howrah, West Bengal, India

Siddhartha Chatterjee MBBS DGO
DNB FRCOG
Director
Calcutta Fertility Mission
Kolkata, West Bengal, India

SM Rahman MD (AIIMS, New Delhi)
Director
Cradle Fertility Centre
Kolkata, West Bengal, India

Sudip Basu MS DNB FRCOG FRCPI
(Ireland) CCT (UK) PG Dip in Gynaecological
USG (CARDIFF, UK) Special Skill Certificate in
USG and assisted reproduction (RCOG, UK)
Consultant Gynecologist and
Subfertility Specialist
Clinical Director
Srishti Clinic
Kolkata, West Bengal, India

Sunita Sharma MD FNB
Senior Consultant
Institute of Reproductive Medicine
Kolkata, West Bengal, India

Sujoy Dasgupta MS DNB MRCOG
Advanced ART Training (Singapore) MSc
(Sexual and Reproductive Medicine, South
Wales, UK)
Consultant Reproductive Medicine
Genome Fertility Centre
Kolkata, West Bengal, India

Suparna Banerjee DGO MD MRCOG
Medical Director
Consultant Gynecologist and
Infertility Specialist
Ankur Fertility Clinic (Kolkata) and
Institute of Reproductive Solution
(Hooghly)
Kolkata, West Bengal, India

From the President's Desk

Dear Fogsians,
Greetings!!

I feel truly blessed and humbled to be installed as 61st President of FOGSI. My presidential theme of this year is "*Swasth Nari, Sukhi Nari*" or "*Healthy Woman, Happy Woman*". The theme is supported by five pillars of Academics, Fellowship, Research, Advocacy and above all Social Work. We aim to focus on academic, social and community health initiatives for the betterment of women health in our country.

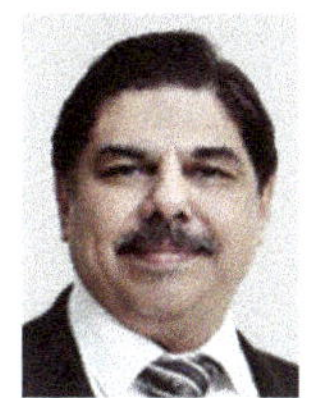

In addition, a new CSR program called *Badlaav*/Change would be launched which is defined by *Integration* of care (Ekikaran), *Equality of treatment* (Samanta) and utilizing *technology* (Takniki) to implement the change. I request you all to stand with me and contribute to these programs which are meant for women upliftment.

Besides these initiatives, I will continue the strong academic activities of the society, as laid down by my predecessors Presidents. Many national and international conferences have been planned throughout the year.

FOGSI has always been committed to deliver various education programs, journals and manuals to help all our fellow members to perform best in their areas of expertise and practice. The AICOG 2023 workshop manuals are a step towards this commitment and are an excellent compilation of all latest advances and day-to-day tips in different fields of obstetrics, gynecology, endoscopy, and infertility. I am sure that these will help all practitioners in keeping themselves abreast of the latest advancements and will also give valuable tips which can be implemented in day-to-day practice.

I congratulate team AICOG and all the editors for their untiring efforts and hard work to write, collate, edit and publish these manuals.

I wish you all a happy reading and a wonderful year full of academics and extracurricular activities.

"I alone cannot change the world, but I can cast a stone across the waters to create many ripples."

–Mother Teresa

Hrishikesh D Pai
President
The Federation of Obstetric and
Gynaecological Societies of India (FOGSI)

Message for the Workshop Manuals

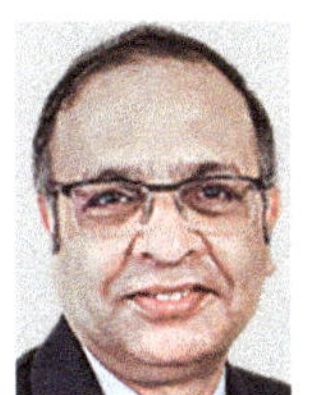

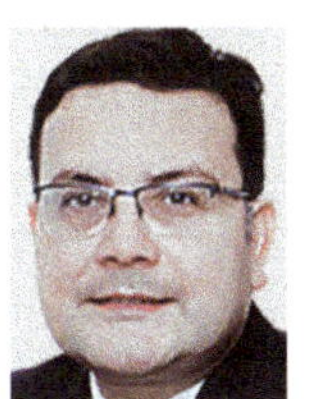

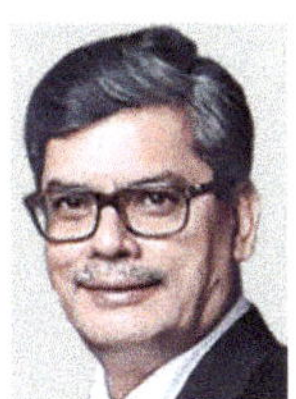

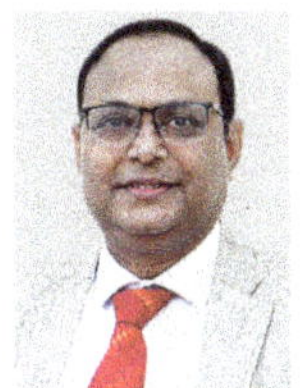

Bhaskar Pal
Organizing
Chairperson

**Basab
Mukherjee**
Organizing
Secretary

**Dibyendu
Banerjee**
Organizing
Secretary

**Kusagradhi
Ghosh**
Chairperson,
Workshop
Committee

Dear Friends,

It is indeed a pleasure to welcome you all to Kolkata for the 65th All India Congress of Obstetrics and Gynecology. The theme '*Creating Tomorrow Together*' has been kept keeping in mind our contemporary approach with a futuristic touch.

The workshop committee has worked diligently over months to offer attending delegates a quality academic extravaganza over a variety of subspecialties to choose from. There are four live workshops covering minimally invasive surgery (basic and advanced), vaginal surgery and fetal interventions. International faculty of repute have been invited to several of the workshops to make them more attractive. We are sure you will enjoy their deliberations and look forward to receiving your feedback for the same.

The workshops at our AICOGs have proven to be active learning hubs and often attracting more crowd than the main scientific program. We know from previous experience that delegates often request for reading material from the event which would be helpful for them to integrate the knowledge harvested from the sessions into their clinical practice.

Partnering with M/s Jaypee Brothers Medical Publishers, we are glad to bring out seven manuals at this AICOG 2023 some of which collate more than one workshop. We sincerely hope these booklets will be of value to you and you will benefit from the same.

We again take this opportunity to wish you all a wonderful time at Kolkata and hope you carry back pleasant memories to last for a long time.

Warm regards!

Contents

Male Infertility—Rational Investigations and Treatment

Sujoy Dasgupta, Sudip Basu

■ INTRODUCTION

Male factors are responsible in 50% cases of subfertility, either as a major factor or a contributory one. Globally the quantity and quality of sperm parameters are declining over last 40 years. The research on "cure" of male infertility is limited because of widespread availability of assisted reproductive technology.

■ SEMEN ANALYSIS

The evaluation of the fertility potential for a man starts with semen analysis. However a single abnormal report does not necessarily indicate infertility in men, because it takes around 64 days' time for the spermatogenesis cycle to complete.

The World Health organization (WHO) in their latest edition, defined the "lower reference ranges" of "normal" semen parameters as the fifth centile.[1] However, men having any parameter below the reference level cannot be termed "infertile", because all the men from whom samples were drawn, became father within one year of regular intercourse.[1] Therefore, what is actually defined as "male infertility" is difficult to answer. To overcome this problem, number of advanced sperm testing has been described, including DNA fragmentation and oxidative stress measurement. However, these tests are not yet standardized and it is not known whether these tests actually improve pregnancy and live birth rate. Therefore, such tests should not be used routinely.[2] Additionally, many laboratories do not comply with the WHO recommendations for semen analysis. Therefore, there is urgent need of training of all the laboratory-staffs doing semen analysis.

Mild Male Infertility

Total motile sperm concentration (TMSC), which is the product of semen volume, total motility and sperm concentration, is more useful to categorize male infertility than individual parameters. TMSC above 10 million is defined as mild male factor problem. In such case, semen analysis should be repeated after 3 months and lifestyle changes are advised (avoidance of smoking, reduction of alcohol use and reduction of weight.[3] Avoidance of scrotal heat by using loose undergarments and avoiding hot bath can be helpful, although convincing evidences are lacking.[3]

Severe Male Infertility

In contrast, in case of severe problems in semen, the analysis should be repeated as soon as possible[3], because there is 25% chance of developing azoospermia over the course of time. Therefore, detailed evaluation is warranted. Additionally, these men should be warned about the risk of developing cardiovascular disease and testicular cancer.[4]

■ EVALUATION

History includes enquiry about use of anabolic steroids, previous surgery and mumps orchitis. The physical examination should not be overlooked especially regarding testicular size (by orchidometer, normal volume 20 cc), location, consistency and presence of vas deferens. It's important to remember that diagnosis of varicocele is always clinical (by Valsalva manoeuvers) and men should not be offered scrotal ultrasound routinely just to diagnose varicocele.

In presence of sperm concentration <10 million/mL, sexual dysfunction or clinical suspicion of endocrinopathy, detailed hormonal evaluation (FSH, LH, testosterone and blood glucose) should be requested. FSH helps to distinguish between hypogonadotrophic hypogonadism (HH, where FSH level will be low) and testicular failure (FSH level high). However, FSH level cannot adequately predict the chance of sperm retrieval in non-obstructive azoospermia (NOA).[4] Testosterone is low in both primary and secondary hypogonadism.[4] In men with anabolic steroid abuse, the testosterone may be elevated with low FSH and LH.

Further evaluation depends on the findings of initial investigations. For suspected obstruction (low volume and acidic semen), transrectal ultrasound (TRUS) should be done. In congenital bilateral absent vas deferens (CBAVD), cystic fibrosis mutation (CFTR) should be checked. Because of the autosomal recessive pattern of transmission, if mutation is detected in the man, the female partner should be tested.[4] Pituitary imaging is required in case of HH. Y chromosome microdeletion test should be offered in severe oligospermia and NOA. In all men with sperm concentration <10 million/mL, karyotype should be offered to diagnose defects in sex chromosomes and some autosomes.[4]

■ MEDICAL MANAGEMENT

Antibiotics: Although leucocytes in semen may indicate male accessory gland infection (MAGI), the exact significance is unknown.[4] Antibiotic should only be prescribed only when there is culture-documented infection.[4] However, antibiotics may not be able to reverse the post-inflammatory anatomical damage caused by the infection.[4]

Antioxidants: High dose of reactive oxygen species (ROS), produced by sperm cells, can cause DNA damage, lipid peroxidation and ultimately infertility. Antioxidants are the molecules which counteract the ROS. The Cochrane review found that antioxidants may increase the pregnancy and live birth rate, although data are of moderate qualities. International guidelines do not support use of antioxidants in idiopathic male infertility.[3,4] Caution should be practiced while advising antioxidants because some amount of oxidative stress is needed for the sperm capacitation.

Gonadotropins: hCG 2000–5000 IU 3 times a week is the treatment of choice in HH.[4] During treatment serum testosterone and the sperm count should be monitored monthly. Sperm parameters become normal within 6–24 months. If hCG alone cannot restore spermatogenesis, FSH is needed (75–150 IU 3 times a week).[4]

Other drugs: The evidences favoring the empirical use of clomiphene and gonadotropins in idiopathic male infertility is not very strong.[3]

In case of low testosterone, exogenous testosterone should not be advised because it can inhibit endogenous gonadotropins, leading to HH. If testosterone (in ng/mL) to estradiol (in pg/mL) ratio is less than 10:1, aromatase inhibitors can be tried.[2,3]

In men with anabolic steroid abuse, stoppage of the drug can restore spermatogenesis, although some may need gonadotropin supplementation.

■ SURGICAL MANAGEMENT

The management of varicocele in men with subfertility is a controversial issue. Varicocelectomy is recommended only in men with grade 3 varicocele, oligospermia and normal female factors, although the level of evidence is "weak".[4] Surgery should not be done in subclinical varicocele and men with normal semen parameters.[4] Even in men with NOA, varicocelectomy leads to appearance of sperms in the semen. Microsurgical varicocelectomy is the most effective method with minimum risks of complications and lower recurrence rates.[4]

For a palpable undescended testis orchidectomy is not advisable because it still produces testosterone. Correction of bilateral cryptorchidism, even in adult, can lead to sperm production in previously azoospermic men.[4] But it's important to perform testicular biopsy at the time of orchidopexy to rule out germ cell neoplasia in situ.

Possibly the best candidates for surgical management are men with ejaculatory duct obstruction (EDO) and previous vasectomy.[4] However, widespread availability of ICSI is responsible for significant decline in surgical skill for correcting varicocele and vas-vas anastomosis.

■ INTRAUTERINE INSEMINATION

Intrauterine insemination (IUI) increases the number of motile and healthy spermatozoa available at the site of fertilization around the time of ovulation.[5] TMSC more than 10 million is associated with significant success in IUI.[5] However, the lower cut-off of TMSC below which IUI should be withheld is not known.[5] There are studies showing that collection of two consecutive ejaculates for IUI can drastically improve the inseminating motile sperm concentration (IMSC), leading to better success rate of IUI. However, there is no evidence that IUI performed twice in a cycle (2 consecutive days) is better than single IUI.[5] There is evidence that IMSC more than 1 million and morphology more than 4% is associated with reasonable success rate in IUI. There is no evidence to suggest any method of sperm preparation over other because all of them are equally useful.[5]

■ IN VITRO FERTILIZATION

In case of TMSC 1–5 million with morphology >4%, conventional in vitro fertilization (IVF) is the treatment of choice.

Indications of ICSI in male infertility are:
- TMSC <1 million
- TMSC <5 million and morphology <4%
- No/poor fertilization in the previous one conventional IVF cycle when TMC <10 million
- No/poor fertilization in the previous two conventional IVF cycles when TMC >10 million
- Surgically retrieved spermatozoa from epididymis or the testes.

Although there is some concern about increased risk of congenital anomaly in the infants born after ICSI, convincing evidence is lacking.

■ SURGICAL SPERM RETRIEVAL

Surgical sperm retrieval (SSR) is the standard way of sperm collection in azoospermia. In obstructive azoospermia (OA), sperms are collected by PESA (percutaneous epididymal sperm aspiration) or MESA (microsurgical epididymal sperm aspiration) and by TESA (testicular sperm aspiration), TESE (testicular sperm extraction) in case of NOA. The live birth rates are significantly lower for NOA than for OA. The cryopreservation of the sperms before ICSI can ensure that sperms are available from that man. Cryopreservation will avoid such unnecessary procedure in the woman and will allow the couple to take the informed decision depending on whether the sperms are obtained or not.

There are some evidences that even in case of non-azoospermic samples, SSR can provide better quality of sperms. It's important to remember that no factors (FSH, testicular size) can accurately predict the chance of sperm retrieval in case of NOA. Only contraindication to SSR is presence of Y chromosome microdeletion involving AZFa and AZFb genes.

■ DONOR SPERM

If ICSI fails or is not affordable by the couple, donor-sperm insemination can be considered depending on the female factor. At least ovulation of the female partner should be assessed before IUI.[3] According to the ART Law, 2022, donors should be recruited and screened by the ART bank only. Notarized affidavit is required for both the donor and the recipient. One donor can donate the sperms only for one recipient in his lifetime.

■ REFERENCES

1. World Health Organization (WHO) 2021. *WHO Laboratory Manual for the Examination and Processing of Human Semen.* 6th ed. Geneva: World Health Organization Press; 2021.
2. Schlegel PN, Sigman M, Collura B, De Jonge CJ, Eisenberg ML, Lamb DJ, Mulhall JP, Niederberger C, Sandlow JI, Sokol RZ, Spandorfer SD, Tanrikut C, Treadwell JR, Oristaglio JT, Zini A. Diagnosis and Treatment of Infertility in Men: AUA/ASRM Guideline PART II. J Urol. 2021 Jan;205(1):44-51. doi: 10.1097/JU.0000000000001520. Epub 2020 Dec 9. PMID: 33295258.
3. NICE Clinical Guideline CG 156. 2013. *Fertility problems: assessment and treatment.* National Institute for Health and Clinical Excellence. Available at https://www.nice.org.uk/guidance/cg1566
4. Jungwirth A, Diemer T, Kopa Z, Krausz C, Minhas S, Tournaye H. (2018) 'EAU Guidelines on Male Infertility'. European Association of Urology. Available at https://d56bochluxqnz.cloudfront.net/media/EAU-Guidelines-on-Male-Infertility-2019.pdf
5. Cohlen B, Bijkerk A, Van der Poel S, Ombelet W. (2018). 'IUI: review and systematic assessment of the evidence that supports global recommendations'. Hum Reprod Update. 24(3):300-319.

Female Genital Tuberculosis: Treatment Protocol for the Infertile

Sunita Sharma, Siddhartha Chatterjee

■ BACKGROUND

Tuberculosis (TB) is a major health concern in developing countries like India and female genital tuberculosis (FGTB) is the commonest form of extrapulmonary TB affecting 5 to 21% of women of reproductive age. FGTB commonly presents with infertility, menstrual dysfunction, and chronic pelvic pain. The prevalence of infertility in FGTB varies from 6–25% in India with a higher incidence in women attending ART clinics. FGTB usually occurs secondary to pulmonary TB and is most often asymptomatic and underdiagnosed, while infertility remains the most common complaint. It is often only suspected during laparoscopy for infertility workup where adhesions and necrotic tissues coupled with tubal obstruction are common findings. FGTB invariably affects the fallopian tubes in 92–100% of cases. Tubal involvement varies from minimal damage causing ectopic pregnancy to extensive damage leading to bilateral complete tubal occlusion. Peritubal adhesion and tubo-ovarian mass have been found in 47.2% of cases. Endometrial involvement is noted in about 35–50% of the cases causing intrauterine adhesion (Asherman's syndrome). Moreover, impaired endometrial receptivity can result in recurrent implantation failure and miscarriages. FGTB may also lead to ovarian damage leading to poor ovarian reserve and chronic anovulation.

Due to improvement of health condition and care the tubercular infection are getting less and less. Instead, tubercular infestation that is mere presence of tubercular bacteria on the genital tract surface is increasing. These sort of infestation often clinically cause latent genital tuberculosis (LGTB). LGTB mostly causes molecular change of the endometrium or tubal surface leading to tubal block, non-receptive endometrium, and diminished ovarian function. LGTB being non infective, passes unnoticed for long time. LGTB may cause local damage which is not that severe. It is observed in the literature that LGTB is associated with tubal block leading to infertility and ectopic pregnancy. Endometrial infestation with MTB may cause unexplained infertility, implantation failure, early embryonic rejection and recurrent miscarriage. The association of LGTB and endometriosis is another cause of concern.

Depending on the virulence of organism and immune response generated by the host, the disease remains either active or becomes asymptomatic with latent infection persisting for many years. Latent infected individuals contain dormant, yet viable bacilli, which may re-activate when the host response becomes low, and as a consequence, the disease may become active again. During the process of reactivation, the bacilli induce immune modulation within the local tissues, which mimics inflammatory reactions. There is a release of harmful cytokines like IL-2, TNF-α, and IFN-γ. The final effect will depend upon how strongly the host tissue (ovarian tissue and endometrium) can resist this trauma. If unable to resist, immune-modulatory impact will affect adversely the endometrial receptivity. Once the adverse impact sets in and ovarian function diminishes, the consequences may continue to persist. Since definite physical symptoms are usually not present, the disease remains undiagnosed or specific investigations are not undertaken to rule out the problem. Due to the paucibacillary nature of the disease, cultures, and smears are often negative. Routine screening tests for pulmonary TB like chest X-ray, tuberculin test, and sputum examination are usually negative.

MANAGEMENT OF INFERTILITY IN FEMALE GENITAL TUBERCULOSIS

Diagnosis: Currently, there is still no single diagnostic test for FGTB, hence a combination of different diagnostic methods should be applied combining clinical suspicion, exhaustive history taking, a comprehensive physical examination, and various test to detect *Mycobacterium tuberculosis* (MTB). In the absence of a perfect diagnostic method, a composite reference standard (CRS) is often advocated for FGTB which consisted of acid-fast bacilli on microscopy or culture, histopathological evidence of epithelioid granuloma, positive GeneXpert on the endometrial sample or definite or probable finding of FGTB on laparoscopy. Polymerase chain reaction (PCR) is a laboratory technique for rapidly producing (amplifying) milllions to billions of copies of a specific segment of DNA, which can then be studied in greater detail. PCR involves using short synthetic DNA fragments called primers to select a segment of the genome to be amplified, and then multiple rounds of DNA synthesis to amplify that segment. This technology is widely available at present commercially where single primer flakes are used. This leads to a low detection rate of only pathogenic tubercle bacilli in humans. Even non-pathogenic bacilli may bring harmful immunomodulation in reproductive organs. To identify a large number of them a multiplex PCR system was developed by Bhattyacharya et al, by modifying three individual PCR to one reaction condition.

Tuberculosis notification: According to the India TB Notification Policy, every health care provider including private practitioners is required to notify the tuberculosis notification portal, Ni-kshay about all TB cases including FGTB.

Medical treatment: Once FGTB is diagnosed, antituberculosis treatment is mandatory. All cases of drug-sensitive TB including patients with irregular treatment or defaulters should be treated with a daily dose of rifampicin, isoniazid, pyrazinamide, and ethambutol for 2 months followed by 4 months of daily therapy of rifampicin, isoniazid, and ethambutol. In drug-resistant FGTB, a longer oral regimen with reserve drugs is given for 18–20 months or a shorter regimen is given for 9–12 months as per WHO and National TB Elimination Program (NTEP) guidelines.

Assisted reproduction: Infertility is the most common presentation in women with FGTB and despite antitubercular therapy, chances of a successful pregnancy are low with increased incidence of ectopic pregnancy and spontaneous abortion. Assisted reproduction remains the most effective treatment option in these women and is advised in patients with blocked fallopian tubes, Asherman's syndrome, or diminished ovarian reserve. As FGTB impairs implantation by reducing endometrial receptivity markers, there is a risk of recurrent implantation failure and a low pregnancy rate even after in vitro fertilization (IVF). In FGTB, poor ovarian response, reduced oocyte quality, and impaired endometrial receptivity usually lead to an unfavorable reproductive outcome, whereas early diagnosis can improve the results. Pregnancy rates in FGTB have been reported to vary from 9% to 28%, and a low live birth rate of <30% along with an increased chance of ectopic pregnancy (10%). Involvement of the uterine cavity with synechiae further worsened the prognosis.

Stem cell-based therapy has gained considerable attention in recent years for treating intrauterine adhesions and Asherman's syndrome. Clinical studies using bone marrow-derived stem cells, mesenchymal stem cells, and autologous menstrual blood-derived stromal cells have been reported in restoring endometrial function and fertility.

Surgical treatment: Surgery is not indicated in FGTB due to associated complications; however, there are a few situations where surgery can be considered before IVF, such as the presence of hydrosalpinx and pyosalpinx, tubo-ovarian masses and abscesses, pelvic adhesions, and Asherman's syndrome.

Tuboplasty should be avoided as it does not improve the chances of pregnancy but increases the risk of ectopic pregnancy and disease flare-up even after antitubercular therapy. Laparoscopy and hysteroscopy are indicated after completion of medical therapy for planning further management of infertility.

Protocols for Treatment of Infertility in Female Genital Tuberculosis

1. First-line management of all diagnosed cases of FGTB is antitubercular therapy.

2. On laparoscopy and hysteroscopy if tubes and uterine cavity appear normal, spontaneous conception can be tried, or ovulation induction drugs given.
3. In case of blocked tubes with normal uterine cavity assisted conception is indicated, clipping of Hydrosalpinx before IVF can improve the conception rate.
4. In case of blocked tubes and mild intrauterine adhesions, hysteroscopic adhesiolysis followed by IVF is advised. Women with severe intrauterine adhesions are advised gestational surrogacy.
5. In case of ovarian failure and severe intra-uterine adhesions, adoption is advised.

◼ CONCLUSION

Genital tuberculosis is one of the main causes of infertility and is usually underdiagnosed due to the asymptomatic nature of the infection and diagnostic challenges. Antitubercular therapy initiated in the early stage of the disease would help to have a better fertility outcome. IVF-ET is a viable option for tubal blockage with normal endometrium with a promising result. Surrogacy and adoption can be recommended if the endometrium and ovaries are damaged.

◼ FURTHER READING

1. Ministry of Health and Family Welfare, Government of India and World Health Organization. INDEX TB Guidelines: guidelines on extra-pulmonary tuberculosis for India. New Delhi: MOHFW; 2016.
2. World Health Organization Guidelines for treatment of drug-susceptible tuberculosis and patient care. Treatment Tuberculosis World Health Organisation, Geneva 2017 Update.
3. Sharma JB, Jain S, Dharmendra S, Singh UB, Soneja M, Kulshrestha V, Vanamail P. An evaluation of Composite Reference Standard (CRS) for diagnosis of Female Genital Tuberculosis, Indian Journal of Tuberculosis, 2022, (In press).
4. World Health Organization (WhO), 2020. WHO consolidated guidelines on tuberculosis: module 4: treatment: drug-resistant tuberculosis treatment. https://apps.who.int/iris/handle/10665/332397.
5. Sharma JB, Sharma E, Sharma S, et al. Recent Advances in Diagnosis and Management of Female Genital Tuberculosis. J Obstet Gynecol India 2021;71: 476-87.
6. Queckbörner S, Davies LC, von Grothusen C, Santamaria X, Simón C, Gemzell-Danielsson K. Cellular therapies for the endometrium: An update. Acta Obstet Gynecol Scand. 2019;98(5):672-77.
7. Chatterjee S, Datta A, Bagchi B, Chatterjee A, et al. Latent genital tuberculosis causes molecular assault on reproduction. AICC RCOG East Zone Bulletin, Special Reproductive Medicine Edition May 21, 2022.

Fibroids with Infertility: A Management Dilemma

Nandita Palshetkar, Fessy Louis, Rohan Palshetkar

INTRODUCTION

Infertility and recurrent miscarriage are associated with fibroids; especially intramural and submucous myomas, which usually cause distortion of the uterine cavity. The basic mechanisms linking fibroids and infertility are diverse, including:

- Distortion of the uterine cavity (fibroid types: 0, 1, 2, 2–5),
- Impaired myometrial/endometrial blood supply,
- Increased uterine contractility,
- Paracrine, hormone and molecular changes,
- A thicker capsule, and
- Defective gene expression [drop in the expression of homeobox A (HOXA)] and endometrial receptivity.

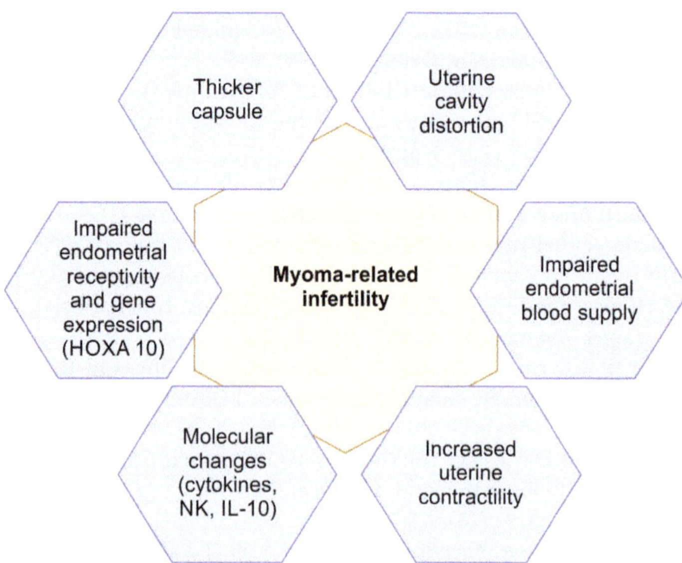

INVESTIGATIONS

Vaginal ultrasound is recommended to identify fibroids, and in making a differential diagnosis of uterine pathologies. Differentiating myomas from adenomyosis can be challenging. In case of doubtful ultrasound findings, magnetic resonance imaging (MRI) can be used to shed more light.

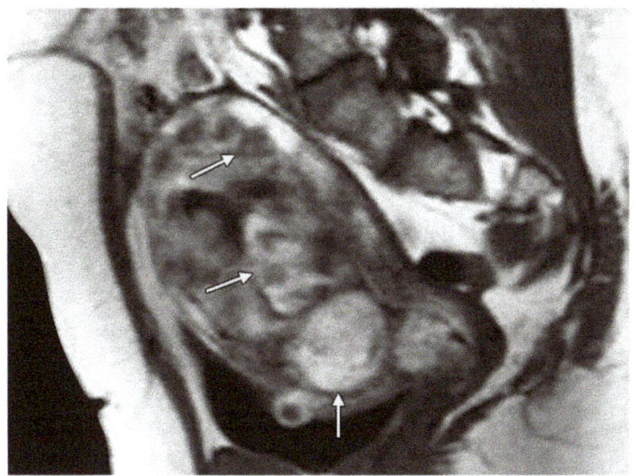

MRI showing multiple fibroids (arrows).

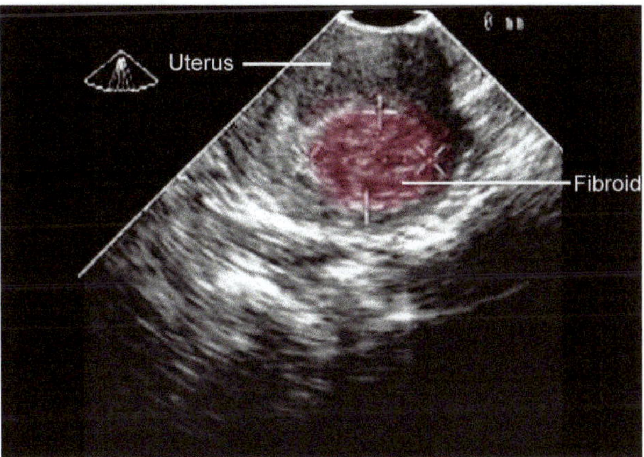

Ultrasound of fibroid (red) in endometrial cavity.

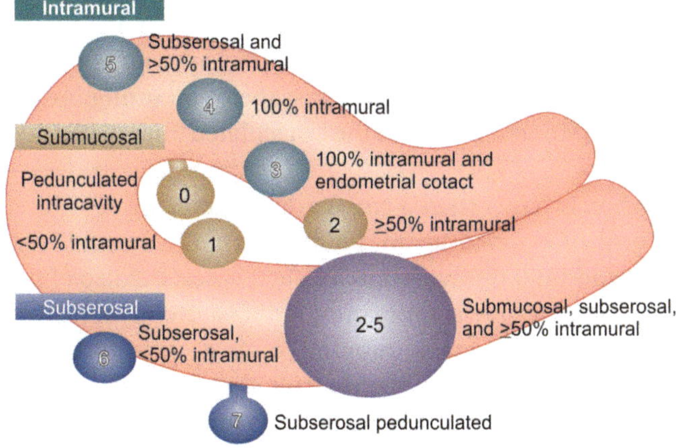

Over the last 10 years, FIGO has distinguished 8 types of myomas; and a hybrid class that accounts for the degree of intramural extension and the distortion of the uterine cavity.

■ MANAGEMENT

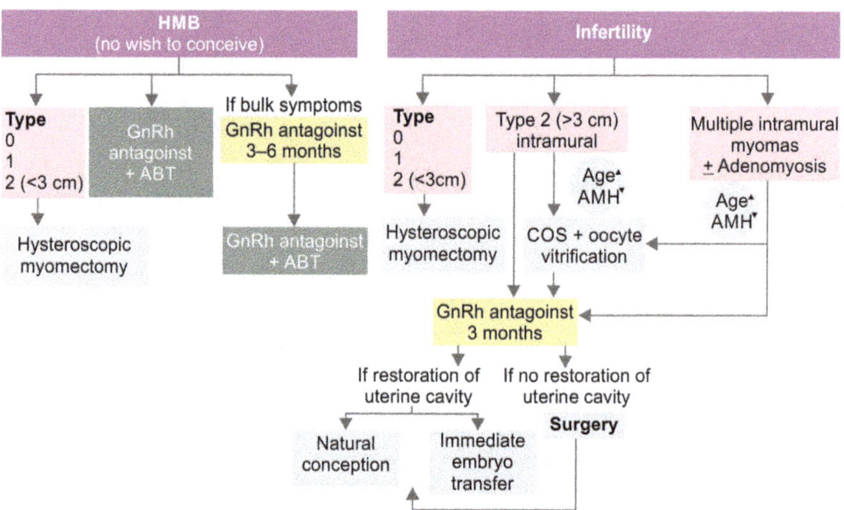

The Current Non-Surgical and Surgical Management Strategies

Conservative non-surgical and surgical approaches include–myomectomy by laparotomy or laparoscopy, myomectomy by hysteroscopy, uterine artery embolization, and other interventions that are performed under radiological or USG guidance.

Hysteroscopic Myomectomy

The advances in recent techniques have highly promoted hysteroscopic myomectomy to the rank of a minimally invasive but standard procedure for submucous fibroids. Small myomas less than 2 cm are mostly removed in an outpatient setting. The slicing technique is the most commonly used approach. Progressive and repeated passage of a cutting loop allows the myoma to be cut into small chips till the fasciculated fibers of the myometrium are visualized.

If the myoma is larger than 3 cm, there is a greater risk of intraoperative complications like perforation or/and damage to the surrounding myometrium and fluid intravasation. In such cases, the use of preoperative GnRH antagonist therapy significantly reduces the myoma size and may facilitate surgery. The residual intramural component rapidly migrates to the uterine cavity after resection of the protruded portion of the myoma which can be resected in a second step or during the same procedure. Hysteroscopic myomectomy has proven to be effective for enhancing fertility, but the failure rate associated with it is usually related to the growth of fibroids in other sites, faulty/incomplete treatment of large intramural (partially submucous) fibroids, or fibroids that are associated with adenomyosis.

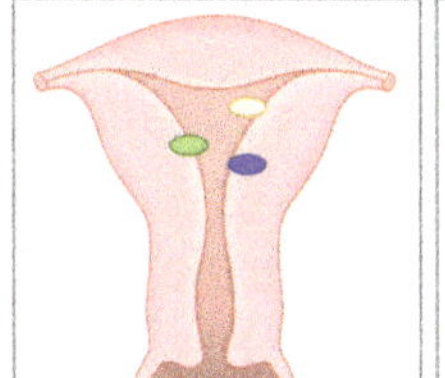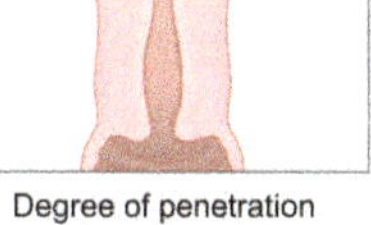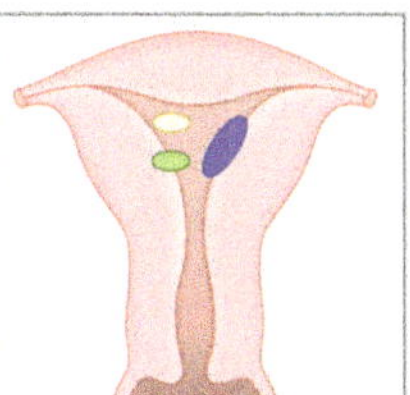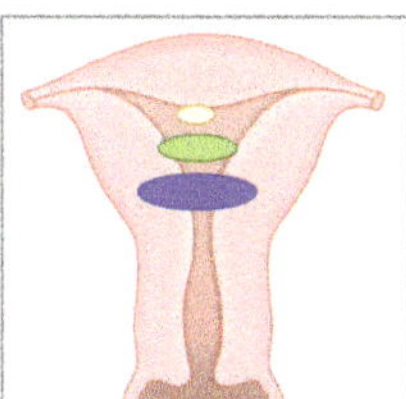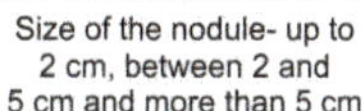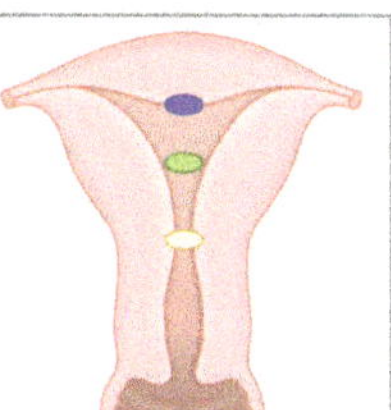

Degree of penetration of the myoma into myometrium	The extension of the base of the nodule with respect to the wall of the uterus	Size of the nodule- up to 2 cm, between 2 and 5 cm and more than 5 cm	Topography- in the lateral wall an extra point is added

STEP-W classification

	Size (cm)	Topography	Extension of the base	Penetration	Lateral wall	Total
0	<2	Low	<1/3	0		
1	2–5	Middle	1/3–2/3	<50%	+1	
2	>5	Upper	>2/3	>50%		

	Score	Group	Complexity and therapeutic options
= Score 0	0–4	I	Low complexity hysteroscopic myomectomy
= Score 1	5–6	II	High complexity hysteroscopic myomectomy. Consider GnRH use. Consider Two-step hysteroscopic myomectomy.
= Score 2	7–9	III	Consider alternatives to the hysteroscopic technique

Infertile patients usually show better clinical pregnancy rates after the resection of submucosal myomas, but the current recommendations for myomectomy are not clear for asymptomatic infertile women with intramural myomas which do not cause distortion of the endometrial lining (FIGO type 3–4), Hence the removal of intramural myomas should be considered in infertile patients seeking ART. The location and size of intramural myomas most likely contribute to the success of ART; so the emphasis should be on the counseling of patients about myomectomy for FIGO type 3 fibroids measuring 2 cm or larger as 1st line therapy.

Laparoscopic Myomectomy

There are well-known shreds of evidence that support the advantages of laparoscopic myomectomy over laparotomy; namely faster recovery with less severe postoperative morbidity, and no major difference between reproductive outcomes after abdominal or laparoscopic myomectomy. Contraindications to laparoscopy include the presence of multiple myomas (≥4) requiring numerous incisions in different sites or with an intramural fibroid measuring more than 10–12 cm in size. During laparoscopy, myomas are removed by mini-laparotomy to avoid the threat of dispersing the friable tissue fragments or with the help of a morcellator inside (or not) a bag or through the pouch of Douglas. The risk of fragment dispersion, with the subsequent parasitic myomas and the appearance of pelvic adenomyotic masses, was first stated in 2006 and still remains a matter of concern that can be avoided with careful removal of all the tissue fragments and extensive peritoneal lavage. On the other hand- the FDA has recently issued warnings about the use of electromechanical power morcellation techniques. However, it should be stressed on the fact that the prevalence of sarcoma in leiomyomas is less than 0.3% and the ongoing debate around the use of electric morcellation has mostly been somewhat inflated, not only owing to the fear of medico-legal issues but also for emotional reasons. The technique of power morcellation in a bag does indeed minimize the overall risk of inadvertent tissue from spreading, but at present, there is no clinical evidence that the technique does not increase the rate of postoperative complications. In some rare cases, histology reveals the presence of a smooth muscle tumor of uncertain malignant potential (STUMP), which also presents as a challenge while taking fertility preservation into consideration.

Over the last 150 years, after the first abdominal myomectomy was reported successful in 1845 by John Atlee and brothers Washington, experts still claim and are debating with regards to the advantages of myomectomy and its vast impact on the reproductive performance of infertile women. The exact localization of the myoma in relation to the junctional zone also plays a crucial role in implantation and deep placentation. Intramural myomas have an adverse impact on reproductive and obstetric outcomes and an improvement in terms of fertility after myomectomy. Concerning the surgical approach and technique, a decision for a laparoscopy as the choice should be balanced between the experience of the surgeon and the uterine pathology, as there is much more to gain for surgeons and patients from a well-performed myomectomy by laparotomy than going ahead with a difficult laparoscopy with inappropriate suturing.

Laparoscopic Thermocoagulation and Cryomyolysis Technique

Laparoscopic cryomyolysis and thermocoagulation both have a similar goal of reducing or suppressing the primary blood flow and inducing myoma shrinkage by causing sclerohyaline degeneration (at very low/high temperatures). For the technique of cryomyolysis, a cryoprobe is used which is inserted into the myoma and cooled to a temperature of less than 90°C. For thermocoagulation, either a monopolar/bipolar probe is used which is placed inside the myoma before delivering an electrical current. The results in terms of success rates of the procedure are very contentious.

Uterine Artery Embolization (UAE)

The technique was first used by Ravina in the year 1995, which triggers ischemic necrosis in myomas; as the myometrium revascularizes. Most myomas are targeted simultaneously. Although UAE is effective for treating most of the symptoms (reduction in myoma size and bleeding), the risk of having a reoperation is still a legitimate concern, reaching rates of 15–20% after a successful embolization and accounting for up to 50% in case of faulty/incomplete infarction. A recent systematic review on pregnancy outcomes after fertility-sparing treatment of uterine fibroids reported a high rate of successful pregnancies (75.6%) after myomectomy, and post-UAE conceptions showed lowest live birth rates of 60.6% and had the highest rates of miscarriage (27.4%). According to a recent paper; fibroid-related quality of life (QoL) two years post-treatment was found to be better in women who underwent myomectomy than those undergoing UAE.

High-Frequency Magnetic Resonance-Guided Focused Ultrasound Surgery (MRgFUS)

The technique uses thermal ablation and MRI to visualize fibroids and to define the target. Ultrasonic energy used is directed at a point inside the myoma which induces coagulative tissue necrosis. In theory- the damage to surrounding tissue is very minimal. However, a recent systematic review by Verpalen et al. has reported poor to moderate quality of evidence on improved symptoms, and the rate of reintervention following the procedure has reached more than 20% in some series.

■ CONCLUSION

Fertility outcomes are found to be decreased in women with submucosal myomas, and removal still seems to confer benefit. Subserosal fibroids on the other hand as such do not affect fertility outcomes, and removal does not confer any such benefits. Intramural myomas however decrease fertility, but the results of various therapies are still unclear. More high-quality evidence-based studies need to be directed to study the value and effectiveness of myomectomy for intramural myomas, with a focus on the issues such as the number, size, and proximity of the myomas to the endometrium.

■ REFERENCES

1. Hum Reprod Update. 2016;22(6):665-86. Published online. 2016;20.
2. Obstet Gynecol Sci. 2018;61(2):192-201. Published online 2018 Feb 13.
3. https://hysteroscopynewsletter.com/2019/01/20/step-w-or-lasmars-classification

Pranay Phukan, Kalpana Udupa

Uterine Anomalies and Subfertility

■ INTRODUCTION

Congenital uterine anomalies (CUAs) results from defective embryological development of the Müllerian ducts. Most CUAs are asymptomatic and are associated with normal reproductive outcomes and some may be associated with adverse reproductive outcomes.

■ PREVALENCE AND ASSOCIATION

A recent meta-analysis has estimated the overall prevalence of CUAs to be 5.5% in an unselected population, 8.0% in infertile women, 13.3% in those with a history of miscarriage and 24.5% in those with miscarriage and infertility.[1] As for the incidence of the specific types, septate and arcuate uterus accounts to 55% of CUAs with the septate uterus being the most common congenital anomaly encountered in clinical practice, while Mayer–Rokitansky–Küster–Hauser (MRKH) syndrome (Müllerian agenesis), seems the rarest.[1]

The association of CUAs with the urinary tract abnormalities is well recognized and up to 40% of patients with a unicornuate uterus and 80% of those with uterus didelphys were found to also have renal anomalies.[2] Furthermore, auditory defects were reported in over 22% of patients with Müllerian anomalies.[2]

■ ETIOLOGY

There are many theories involving genetic, environmental, and pharmacologic factors and the role of genetic factors remains unclear. Normal karyotyping was found in 92% of women with Müllerian anomalies and 7.7% of these women had abnormal karyotypes.

Several genes have been implicated in the development of Wolffian and Müllerian ducts (e.g., Pax2, Pax8, Lim1 and Emx2).[1] Conversely, the BCL2 gene (which is involved with regulating apoptosis) has been implicated in the persistence of the uterine septum, suggesting the role of apoptosis as

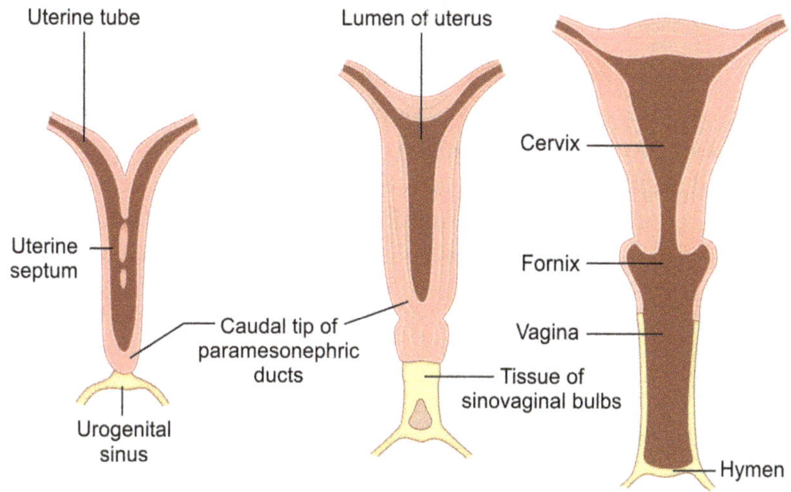

Fig. 1: Embryonic formation of female reproductive system.

a potential mechanism by which regression of the uterine septum takes place.

During early pregnancy, exposure to extra-uterine and intra-uterine environmental factors, such as ionizing radiation (e.g., x-rays and y-rays), intrauterine infections (e.g., rubella) or drugs with teratogenic effects (e.g., thalidomide and diethylstilbestrol), has been implicated in the causation of fetal genital tract defects.

There are three phases **(Fig. 1)** of Müllerian duct development and defective development at any of these phase results in development of CUAs.

1. Organogenesis defects—agenesis or hypoplasia (e.g., absent uterus and unicornuate uterus).
2. Fusion of both Müllerian ducts
   a. Horizontal fusion or unification defects—partial fusion or unification defect (e.g., bicornuate uterus) or complete fusion or unification defect (uterine didelphys).
   b. Vertical fusion defects—imperforate hymen or a transverse vaginal septum.
3. Septa resorption or canalization defects—complete septate uterus, partial septate uterus, or arcuate uterus.

■ CLASSIFICATION

Several classifications of uterine malformations were suggested over the years. The system of American Fertility Society (AFS—1988), now known as the American Society for Reproductive Medicine (ASRM), was the most widely used classification over past three decades, but it was introduced without morphometric criteria, making differentiation between anomalies difficult.

One of the most recent classifications **(Fig. 2)** was developed jointly by the European Society of Human Reproduction and Embryology (ESHRE) and the European Society for Gynecological Endoscopy (ESGE) in 2013, through a structured Delphi procedure. It includes descriptions for all female genital tract malformations—not solely uterine. Cervical and vaginal anomalies are classified in independent supplementary subclasses. An arcuate uterus, although the mildest form of resorption failure, is not considered as clinically relevant and is not included in this classification.

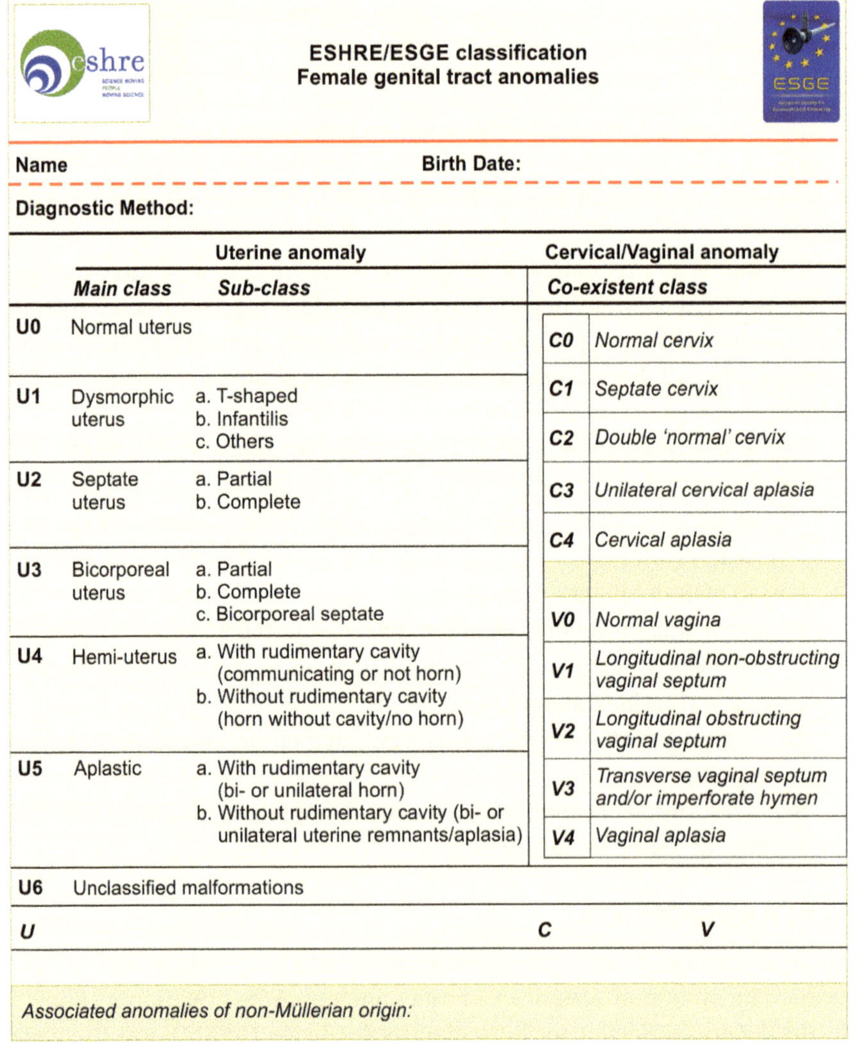

ESHRE/ESGE classification
Female genital tract anomalies

Name **Birth Date:**

Diagnostic Method:

Uterine anomaly			Cervical/Vaginal anomaly	
Main class	*Sub-class*		*Co-existent class*	
U0 Normal uterus			*C0*	*Normal cervix*
U1 Dysmorphic uterus	a. T-shaped b. Infantilis c. Others		*C1*	*Septate cervix*
			C2	*Double 'normal' cervix*
U2 Septate uterus	a. Partial b. Complete		*C3*	*Unilateral cervical aplasia*
			C4	*Cervical aplasia*
U3 Bicorporeal uterus	a. Partial b. Complete c. Bicorporeal septate		*V0*	*Normal vagina*
U4 Hemi-uterus	a. With rudimentary cavity (communicating or not horn) b. Without rudimentary cavity (horn without cavity/no horn)		*V1*	*Longitudinal non-obstructing vaginal septum*
			V2	*Longitudinal obstructing vaginal septum*
U5 Aplastic	a. With rudimentary cavity (bi- or unilateral horn) b. Without rudimentary cavity (bi- or unilateral uterine remnants/aplasia)		*V3*	*Transverse vaginal septum and/or imperforate hymen*
			V4	*Vaginal aplasia*
U6 Unclassified malformations				
U			*C*	*V*

Associated anomalies of non-Müllerian origin:

Fig. 2: *(Contd...)*

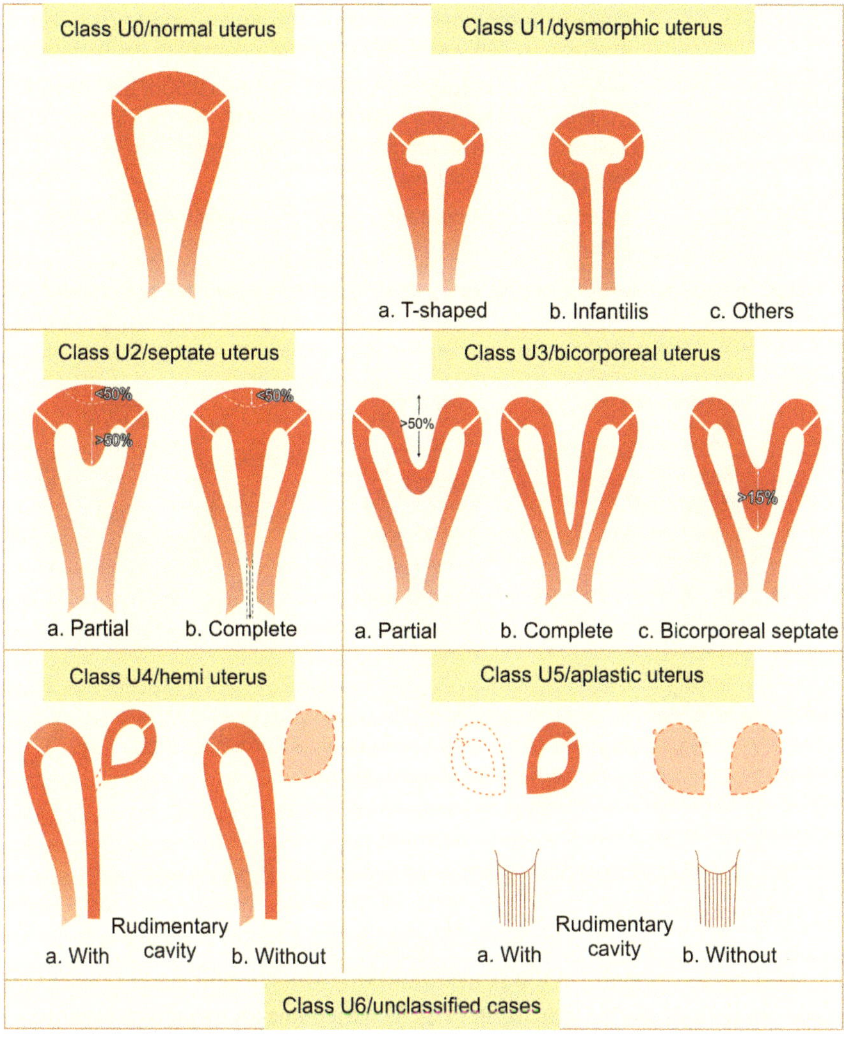

Fig. 2: ESHRE/ESGE classification of female genital tract anomalies (2013).

Controversies in the Classification (Fig. 3)

One of the most prominent issues in the classification is regarding septate uterus. It lacks a universally accepted definition of this condition. In 2016, the ASRM updated its classification of uterine septum (ASRM–2016)[3] and officially endorsed morphometric criteria for distinguishing between septate, normal/arcuate and bicornuate uterus (different to that proposed by ESHRE/ESGE).

Normal/arcuate—depth from interstitial to apex of indentation less than 1 cm and angle of indentation more than 90°.

ASRM 2016	Internal fundal indentation depth:1.5 cm and angle of internal indentation <90° and external fundal indentation depth <1 cm
ESHRE/ESGE 2016	Internal fundal/uterine indentation depth >50% of uterine wall thickness and external indentation depth <50% of uterine wall thickness, with uterine wall thickness measured above inter-ostial/inter-cornual line
CUME 2018	Internal fundal indentation depth c:1 cm and external fundal indentation depth <1 cm

Fig. 3: Septate uterus according to ESHRE/ESGE, ASRM and CUME definitions.[4]

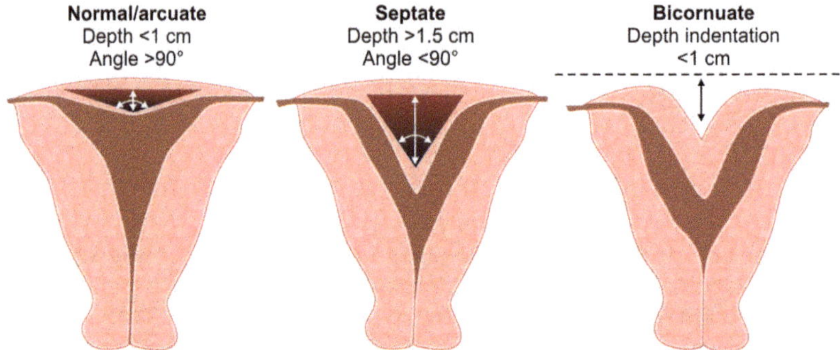

Fig. 4: Diagrams of the ASRM definitions of normal/arcuate, septate, and bicornuate uterus.

Septate—depth of interstitial line to apex more than 1.5 cm and angle of indentation less than 90°.

Bicornuate—external fundal indentation more than 1 cm **(Fig. 4)**.

Recently, ASRM (2021)[3] has modified the AFS classification (1988) and come up with a new classification **(Fig. 5)** which has pictorial representation of anomalies. The advantages of the classification are simplicity, recognizability and correlation with clinical pregnancy outcome.

■ REPRODUCTIVE IMPLICATIONS[1]

Congenital uterine anomalies are mostly diagnosed incidentally during investigations for subfertility, recurrent miscarriage, or menstrual disorders (dysmenorrhea). Women with agenesis (MRKH syndrome or segmental hypoplasia) present with primary amenorrhea. Obstructive uterine anomalies (unicornuate uterus with a rudimentary horn, uterine didelphys with obstructed hemivagina or vaginal/cervical agenesis) present with pelvic pain secondary to hematometra, hematocolpos or endometriosis. Uterine anomalies with longitudinal vaginal septa present most commonly with dyspareunia or occasionally menstrual abnormalities. Septate uterus causes infertility or recurrent pregnancy loss (RPL) by providing a suboptimal site for implantation, disorderly and decreased blood supply insufficient to support placentation and embryo growth, and uncoordinated uterine contractions or reduced uterine capacity. Uterine anomalies have been implicated as potential causes of infertility, recurrent miscarriages, preterm delivery, fetal malpresentation and fetal growth restriction. These women are also reported to have increased rates of pre-eclampsia and stillbirth.[1]

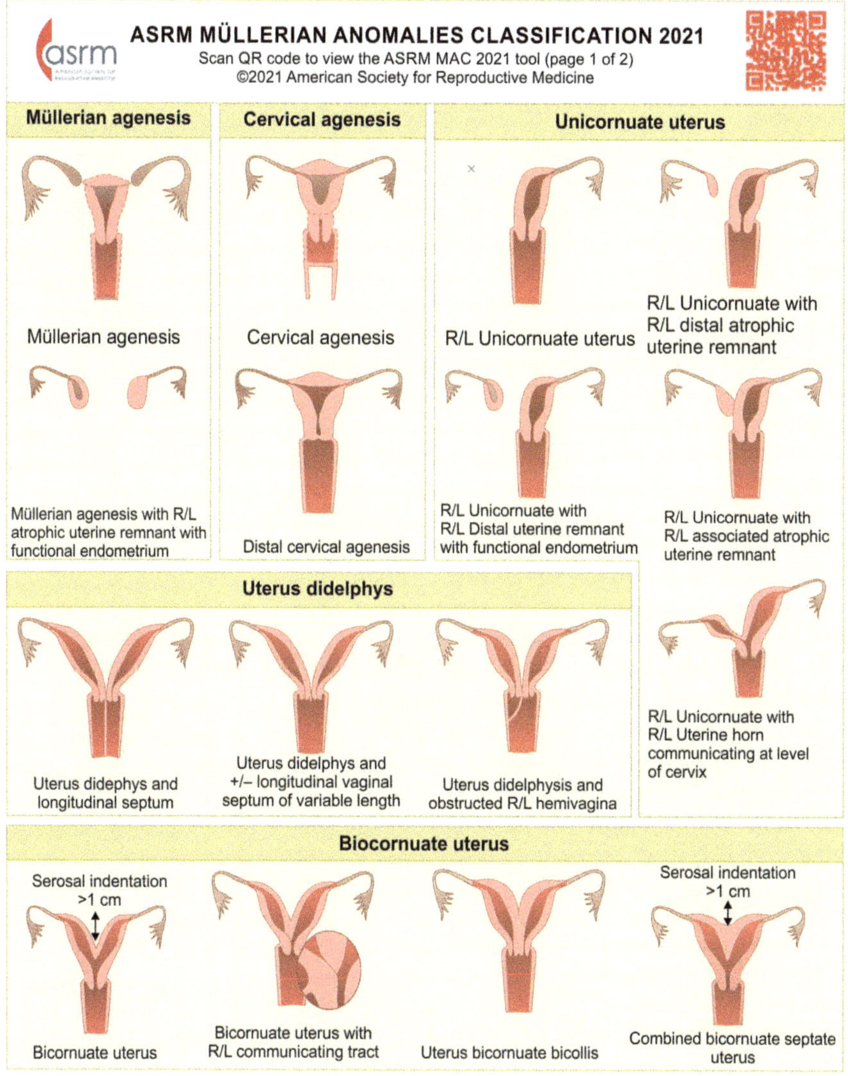

Fig. 5: *(Contd...)*

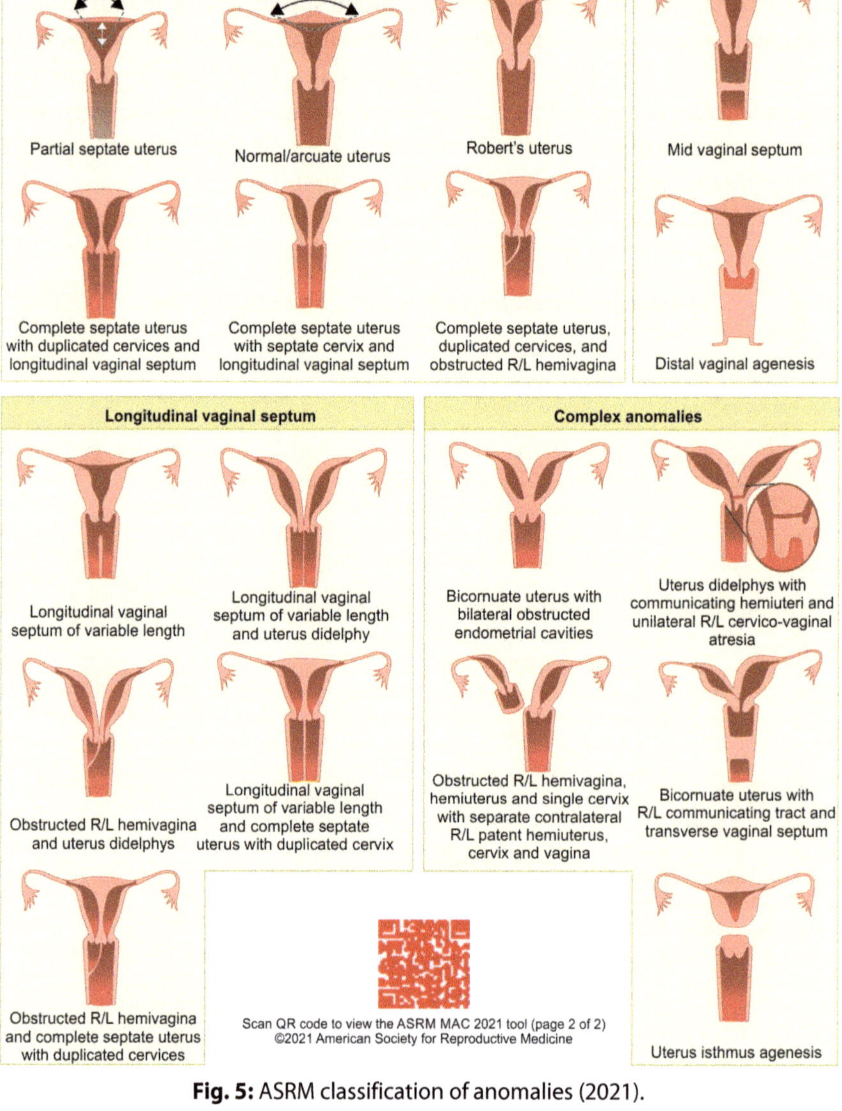

Fig. 5: ASRM classification of anomalies (2021).

◼ DIAGNOSIS

Clinical examination Hysterosalpingography (HSG) 2-D ultrasound

3-D Ultrasound: Hystero-contrast-salpingography (HyCoSy) Magnetic Resonance Imaging (MRI) Laparoscopy & Hysteroscopy

Karyotyping: Recommendations (consensus between CONUTA group members and invited experts)

- The combination of gynecological examination and 2D US is recommended as the current standard for the evaluation of asymptomatic women

'Symptomatic' or high risk can be used to describe the following groups presenting with clinical problems that could be associated with the presence of female genital anomalies and expected to have higher prevalence than that of the general population.

Diagnostic Workup in Symptomatic Group

3D Ultrasound (US) (vaginal) is recommended as the 'reference standard' for diagnosis of female genital anomalies, supplemented by MRI and endoscopic evaluation as 'reference standards' in complex cases (defined as anomalies resulting from disturbances in more than one stage of normal embryological development and including deviations in more than one organ of the female genital tract) or in diagnostic dilemmas.[1]

Diagnostic Workup in Adolescents

Adolescents with symptoms suggestive for the presence of a female genital should be evaluated with Gynecological examination, abdominal and/or transrectal 2D US and 3D US. MRI is considered as a 'first line' diagnostic procedure for those patients.

A urinary tract ultrasound scan, MRI or intravenous pyelogram should be recommended in all women diagnosed with a CUA.

■ MANAGEMENT OPTIONS

The aims of CUA management are to treat anatomical distortions associated with obstructive anomalies, to relieve symptoms, to improve quality of life and to avoid long-term health and reproductive adverse consequences; and for non-obstructive anomalies, to improve reproductive outcomes in infertile women or women who have experienced recurrent miscarriages.

Obstructive anomaly: Unicornuate uterus usually does not warrant surgical intervention, but functioning rudimentary uterine horns, frequently associated with unicornuate uterus, needs surgical removal to prevent the risk of hematometra or pregnancy occurring in the horn.

Non-obstructive Anomalies

Bicornuate and Didelphic Uteri (Unification or Fusion Defects)

Traditionally, abdominal metroplasty was performed to and it remains as the only surgical treatment available for women with bicornuate or didelphic uteri. However, it is associated with higher risks of complications and is not considered or advised in the absence of significant adverse reproductive history.

Septate Uterus

The uterine septum may be repaired with a laparotomy (Jones or modified Tompkin's procedures) or with hysteroscopic techniques. The current treatment of choice for septate uterus is hysteroscopic metroplasty or hysteroscopic transcervical division of the uterine septum. Several observational studies indicate that hysteroscopic septum incision is associated with improved clinical pregnancy rates in women with infertility.

Adhesion prevention: Post procedure intrauterine adhesion is an expected complication and most commonly used preventive measures are intrauterine contraceptive device [IUCD]-after removal of copper thread, hormonal treatment with estrogen, combination therapy with IUCD and hormonal treatment, placement of an intrauterine balloon for 5 days and intrauterine auto-cross linked hyaluronic acid gel.

Re-evaluation by second-look hysteroscopy at 1–3 months postoperatively, can be offered to evaluate adhesion formation and any residual septum.[3]

■ CONCLUSION

Not all women with CUA are infertile. There is an association between infertility and CUA and has impact on reproductive outcome. As of now, there is no uniformly accepted and perfect classification system of CUAs available. Most CUAs are not suitable/amenable to surgery. Some patients with septate uterus may benefit from a well performed hysteroscopic metroplasty. Thorough investigations for co-existent pathology must be performed. All the women with uterine anomaly and those treated with hysteroscopic resection of uterine septum should be followed up by 12 weeks, using an appropriate preterm birth care pathway as outlined in UK Preterm Birth Clinical Network Guidance.

■ REFERENCES

1. Chan YY, Jayaprakasan K, Zamora J, Thornton JG, Raine Fenning N, Coomarasamy A. The prevalence of congenital uterine anomalies in unselected and high risk populations: a systematic review. Hum Reprod Update. 2011;17: 76171.
2. Oppelt P, von Have M, Paulsen M, Strissel PL, Strick R, Brucker S, et al. Female genital malformations and their associated abnormalities. Fertil Steril. 2007;87(2):335-42.
3. The American Fertility Society. The American Fertility Society classifications of adnexal adhesions, distal tubal occlusion, tubal occlusion secondary to tubal ligation, tubal pregnancies, Müllerian anomalies and intrauterine adhesions. Fertil Steril. 1988;49:944-55.
4. Practice Committee of the American Society for Reproductive Medicine. Uterine septum: a guideline. Fertil Steril. 2016;106:530-40.
5. Ludwin A, Martins WP, Nastri CO, Ludwin I, Coelho Neto MA, Leitão VM, et al. Congenital Uterine Malformation by Experts (CUME): better criteria for distinguishing between normal/arcuate and septate uterus? Ultrasound Obstet Gynecol. 2018;51:101-9.

How to Solve a Problem like Polycystic Ovary Syndrome: Initial Steps

Suparna Banerjee

■ INTRODUCTION

Polycystic ovary syndrome (PCOS) is a chronic endocrine and metabolic disorder characterized by dysfunctional ovulation, androgen excess and/or sonographic appearance of polycystic ovaries. Prevalence of PCOS varies depending on the criteria to make the diagnosis and it varies with ethnicity. Though it is a worldwide health issue for women but sometimes it is under appreciated. The prevalence of PCOS can be as high as 15%–20% when European society of Human reproduction and Embryology/American society of reproductive medicine criteria are used. Indian prevalence of PCOS in between 8.2%–22.5% depending on the diagnostic criteria used

■ MORPHOLOGICAL CLASSIFICATION OF POLYCYSTIC OVARY SYNDROME

Type A	Type B
• High androgens/symptoms • Irregular periods/ovulation • Polycystic ovaries	• High androgens/symptoms • Irregular periods/ovulation • Normal ovaries

Type C	Type D
• High androgens/symptoms • Regular periods (<35 days) • Polycystic ovaries	• Normal androgens • Irregular periods/ovulation • Polycystic ovaries

Polycystic ovary syndrome not only cause menstrual irregularities and infertility but it also causes long term health problems like Prediabetes, type two Diabetes, dyslipidemia, hypertension, cardiac problems, endometrial carcinoma, sleep apnea and depression. Thus it is very important to diagnose the problem early to prevent the long term consequences.

■ PATHOPHYSIOLOGY OF POLYCYSTIC OVARY SYNDROME

Polycystic ovary syndrome was first described by Stein and Leventhal in 1935. Since then so many years passed, but etiology remains unclear. But it is the most common endocrinopathy which affects women and a leading cause for infertility.

The key pathology is insulin resistance and Androgen excess. Largescale studies suggest genetic relationship of it.

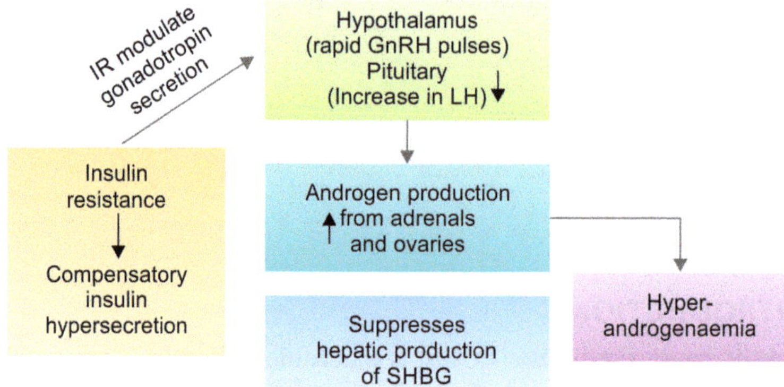

RISK FACTORS FOR POLYCYSTIC OVARY SYNDROME

- Obesity in childhood and adolescence.
- Low birth weight baby with premature menarche who gained excessive weight at puberty.
- Presence of Acanthosis Nigricans
- Family history of Diabetes from maternal side.

HOW DO WOMEN WITH POLYCYSTIC OVARY SYNDROME PRESENT?

- *Irregular cycles:* sometimes amenorrhea and only withdrawal bleeding or delayed cycles and sometimes heavy bleeding after a period of amenorrhea. For them other causes of menstrual disorders like Hypo-thyroidism, Hyperprolactinemia or endometrial hyperplasia/polyp to be excluded. As menstrual disorder is very common after Menarche, two years to be waited for maturation of Hypothalamo–Pituitary-Ovarian axis before marking them as PCOS. But if menstrual interval is more than ninety days , irrespective of years after menarche, it is a sign of PCOS. They can also be present as primary amenorrhea.
- *Hirsutism:* excessive facial coarse hair, body hair and acne.
- Acanthosis Nigricans and cliteromegaly.
- Obesity
- Infertility
- Non-alcoholic fatty liver disease.

DIAGNOSIS OF POLYCYSTIC OVARY SYNDROME

Sonographic evaluation of ovaries and uterus in post menstrual phase (dominant follicle/corpus luteum gives higher ovarian volume). Ovarian volume >12.0 cm^3 echogenic stroma, more than twenty antral follicles per ovary by Trans vaginal ultrasonography.

Ultrasound Evaluation of Abdomen to Rule Out Androgen Secreting Tumor to be Done

Blood tests like: Oral Glucose Tolerant test with seventy five grams of glucose (ASRM and Androgen Excess Society recommendation), Lipid profile, Thyroid function test, complete hemogram to be done for all PCOS women. Serum total testosterone or free testosterone level , serum seventeen hydroxy progesterone and DHEAS can be done to rule out adrenal androgen secretion. But these androgen tests are not mandatory for diagnosis. Clinical signs of hyperandrogenism are the key for diagnosis. Serum anti-müllerian hormone estimation is not required to diagnose PCOS and even for infertile women if we have already diagnosed her as PCOS, we should not use this expensive test as a routine.

Serum SHBG level is usually low for PCOS, but this test should not be done routinely. HOMA score for assessing Insulin resistance is not to be done routinely.

■ TREATMENT

Lifestyle intervention is the key management for PCOS at all ages. As Insulin resistance and disorder of carbohydrate metabolism is present in PCOS, even non-obese or lean PCOS women also get benefit from it. Low carbohydrate diet rich in fibers and protein with exercise for forty five minutes to one hour is absolutely essential. Weight reduction improves Insulin resistance and decreases androgen concentration. As a result, these interventions regularize menstrual cycle, induce ovulation and prevent long term co-morbidities like Diabetes and dyslipidemia. Clinical practice guidelines for Endocrine society suggest life style modification is the first line management for prevention of cardiovascular disease for PCOS. Healthy diet and weight reduction also help to prevent NASH (Non-alcoholic steatohepatitis).

Younger women or women who are not planning pregnancy **combined oral contraceptive pills** can regularize their cycle, reduce menstrual blood loss and give them effective contraception. Combined contraceptives lowers free androgen level by increasing SHBG level and as it provides regular withdrawal bleeding; it prevents endometrial hyperplasia due to long periods of amenorrhea. Among contraceptive pills antiandrogen cyproterone acetate or antimineralocorticoid drosperinone containing pills are better choice for this group of women as these lowers the free androgen level and thus helps in improving acne and hirsutism. Oral contraceptive pill increases the risk of deep vein thrombosis thus risk assessment is necessary before prescribing oral contraceptive pill, especially for long term use.

For very young girls **only progesterone pills** can be given for their withdrawal bleeding to protect their endometrium from ill effect of unopposed Estrogen.

Metformin, a biguanide, is used for management of altered carbohydrate metabolism. For PCOS it is very effective as it reduces insulin resistance, which is the key factor for this problem. Metformin also reduced hyperandrogenism, so chance of ovulation increases. But for ovulation induction its monotherapy is not recommended. If glucose intolerance is not established with investigation, routine Metformin treatment is not recommended specially for young age group. Metformin can be used as second line therapy for prevention of cardiovascular disease and reduction of weight. (ESHRE recommendation)

Use of **Inositol** in any form can be helpful for PCOS management, but ESHRE recommends it as an experimental therapy.

For management of an ovulatory infertility for PCOS ovulation induction is done with oral ovulogens. **Letrozole** is the first line therapy for ovulation induction according to ESHRE. The reason behind that is likelihood of ovulation, pregnancy rate and live birth rate, all are slightly higher than Clomiphene citrate. Risk of multi fetal pregnancy is lower, and hot flush like side effects are not present for Letrozole. It can be used in clomiphene resistance cases. Letrozole resistance is very rare.

Clomiphene citrate can still be used as ovulogen for PCOS. Metformin can be added for obese PCOS with clomiphene, especially where clomiphene has failed to induce ovulation in an effective dose.

Gonadotropins are recommended as second line therapy for ovulation induction in PCOS especially where no other factors for infertility are present and where oral ovulogens have been already tried without success. Risk of using this is chance of multifetal pregnancy is high. As cost of therapy increases significantly, counseling must be done before starting this therapy. Effective ultrasound monitoring, availability of gonadotropins, affordability of patients to be considered before starting this treatment. Low dose protocol should be done to optimize monofollicular development. There is no evidence that one type of gonadotropin is better than other. Gonadotropin induced ovulation should only be triggered if less than three mature follicles are present.

Laparoscopic ovarian drilling can be offered as second line therapy for an ovulatory PCOS who are also resistant to clomiphene, as is can induce monofollicular ovulation later. But risk of intra and post-operative complications to be bear in mind. Cost and complication due to operation should be counseled properly.

When gonadotropin treatment combined with intra-uterine insemination is unsuccessful, IVF or in vitro fertilization should be offered.

Bariatric surgery can be an option for severely obese PCOS who are not able to reduce weight, the cost of the operation and risk of the procedure should be thoroughly counseled.

■ FURTHER READING

1. ACOG Practice Bulletin No. 108. 2009 (reaffirmed 2013). PCOS Clinical Management Guidelines for Obstetricians and Gynecologists.
2. ESHRE Guideline: International Evidence-based guidelines for the assessment and management of PCOS 2018.
3. Stein IF, Leventhal NL. Amenorrhea associated with bilateral polycystic ovaries. Am J Obstet Gynecol. 1935;29:181-191.
4. Thessaloniki and ESHRE/ASRM-Sponsored PCOS consensus workshop group (2008).

Intrauterine Insemination: Easy Protocol for Beginners

Rishma Dhillon Pai, Jyotsana Singh

INTRODUCTION

Intrauterine insemination (IUI) with or without controlled ovarian stimulation (COS) is a simple and inexpensive procedure for treating sub fertility in women with patent tubes, male factor (sexual dysfunction, retrograde ejaculation), cervical/vaginal factor, immunological factor, chronic anovulation and unexplained infertility.

Studies have shown IUI gives better results when it follows COS rather than natural cycle IUI or planned intercourse.[1]

INDICATIONS FOR OVULATION INDUCTION IN INTRAUTERINE INSEMINATION

Ovulation inducing drugs can be used in patients with anovulatory cycles which consists of

1. Group 1: Hypogonadotropic hypogonadism (hypothalamus and pituitary failure)
2. Group 2: Hypothalamic pituitary dysfunction (PCOS)
3. Group 3: Ovarian failure.

Numerous drugs most commonly used for ovulation induction in IUI are:

1. Clomiphene citrate
2. Letrozole
3. Gonadotropin
4. Clomiphene citrate with gonadotropin
5. Letrozole with gonadotropin
6. Gonadotropin with GnRH antagonist
7. Clomiphene citrate/Letrozole with gonadotropin with GnRH antagonist.

OVULATION INDUCING AGENTS AND PROTOCOLS FOR INTRAUTERINE INSEMINATION

1. *Clomiphene citrate:* It is a selective estrogen receptor modulator which is one of the most commonly used drugs to induce ovulation in women with oligo and anovulatory cycles. It is used in a dose of 50 mg to 150 mg daily from (Day 2/3 of periods) for 5 days.

It gives an ovulation rate of about 60–85% and clinical pregnancy rate/cycle of about 10–20%.[2]

It acts as a partial estrogen agonist in the hypothalamus causing estrogen negative feedback inhibition, thereby resulting in increased deliverance of gonadotrophins, thereby leading to folliculogenesis.

Low pregnancy rates may be due to antiestrogenic effects on cervical mucous and reduced endometrial blood flow and thickness.

2. *Letrozole:* A non-steroidal aromatase inhibitor which competitively inhibits aromatase enzyme thereby preventing conversion of androgen to estrogen. It has been successfully used for ovulation induction in PCOS patients with good pregnancy outcomes and decreased multiple gestation.[3] It is typically prescribed in a dose of 2.5 mg to 5 mg per day for 5 days starting from day 2/3 of the cycle. Letrozole shows favorable and increased stromal blood flow with thicker endometrium thereby more favorable for implantation and pregnancy compared to CC.

   Extended letrozole therapy for ovulation induction in CC resistant women with PCOS: In this 2.5 mg of letrozole is given daily starting day 1 of menses for 10 days. This protocol proves to be more efficient with more mature follicles and more clinical pregnancy without risk of OHSS and multiple pregnancy.

   Letrozole step up protocol: In this one, two, three and four tablets of letrozole 2.5 mg daily is given on menstrual cycle day 2,3,4, and 5 respectively. It was noted that no of growing follicles. (>15 mm) on the day of HCG administration was more than compared to CC.

3. *Gonadotropins:* Had shown supremacy to CC and letrozole in improving clinical outcomes of IUI.

The elements which affect the dose and type of gonadotropin to be used are (a) age (b) BMI (c) ovarian reserve and (d) dose needed for stimulation in previous cycle.

Regimens:

a. *Conventional:* A daily dose of 75–150 units of gonadotropin is started from day 2/3 followed by follicular scan and serum E2 levels performed from day 8 onwards. It gives a clinical pregnancy rate up to 30%, however risk of hyperstimulation and multiple pregnancy is high. This protocol may be used in older patients or poor responders.

b. *Low dose step up regimen:* A low dose of 37.5–75 units/day is given and a step wise subsequent dose is increased if required with the aim of getting single dominant follicle and to avoid OHSS and multiple pregnancy. This regimen is particularly helpful for PCOS patients.

   If E2 >200 pg/mL on D8 or follicle size is >10 mm same dose is continued, if both are inadequate the dose is stepped up by 37.5 units/day every week.

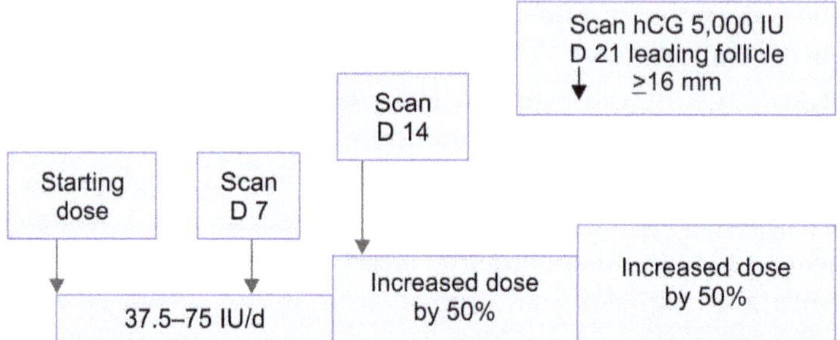

c. *Step down regimen:* A daily dose of 150 units of gonadotropin is started on Day 2 and continued till dominant follicle of >10 mm is observed. After this the dose is decreased to 112.5 Units per day for 3 days followed by 75 units per day for next 3 days.

Clomiphene Citrate vs. Letrozole with Gonadotropin

- *Clomiphene citrate with gonadotropin:* A daily dose of 100 mg of CC from D2–D6 and inj FSH/HMG 75 units or 150 units given on D6 and D8.

- *Letrozole with gonadotropin:* A daily dose of 5 mg of Letrozole from D2 to D6 and inj FSH/HMG of 75/150 units given on D6 and 8 of menstrual cycle.

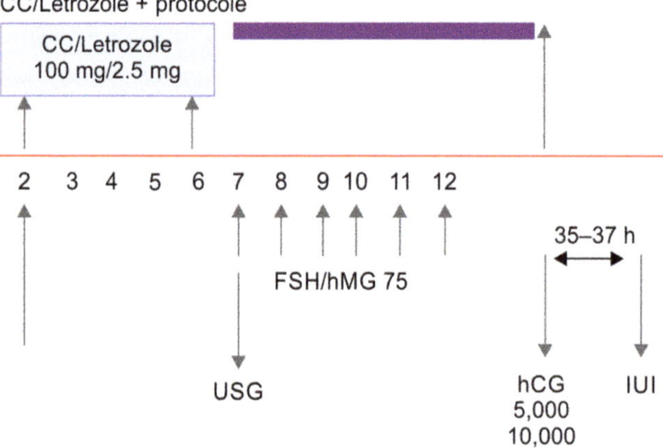

The clinical pregnancy rate is higher in Letrozole group due to antiestrogenic effect of CC on endometrium and cervical mucous. OHSS is more predominant in CC treated patients.[3] The number of mature follicles is not significantly different between the two groups.

d. *GnRH antagonist in IUI:* Acts by competitive inhibition of GnRH receptors which result in decline of FSH/LH levels and preventing premature LH surge. It can be given in single dose or daily dose regimen in follow:

- *Lubeck protocol:* Antagonist is given daily in a dose of 0.25 mg subcutaneous (s.c) from day 6 (fixed protocol) or when follicle size reaches 14 mm (flexible protocol) till the day of HCG administration.[4]

- *French protocol:* Antagonist are started as a single dose 3 mg when serum E2 level is about 150–200 pg/mL and follicle size reaches 14 mm.[5]

Both the protocols are equally effective.

■ TRIGGER IN INTRAUTERINE INSEMINATION

1. HCG in IUI—5000 or 10,000 IU of HCG is administered once the leading follicle is more than or equal to 18 mm and IUI is performed after approximately 36 hrs.
2. GnRH agonist in IUI—0.1 mg single dose is administered followed by IUI after 36 hrs.

Despite the fact that HCG is widely used for final oocyte maturation, it's prolonged luteotrophic effects may lead to development of OHSS so GnRH agonist is more often used in patients who are prone to develop OHSS (like PCOS patients).

■ REFERENCES

1. Intrauterine insemination fundamentals revisited; Gautam N Allahabadia; JOGS of India. 2017;385-92.
2. Clomiphene citrate vs. Letrozole with GnRH in IUI cycles: Int J Reproductive Bio med. 2017;15:49-54.
3. Mitwally Mf, Said T, Galal A, et al. Letrozole step up protocol. Fertilsteril. 2008;S23-4.
4. Mitwally MF, Casper RF. Aroma tase inhibition in ovulation induction in women with PCOS; Reprod technology. 2000;10:244-7.
5. Mitwally MF, CaSperRF. Use of an aromatase inhibitor for induction of ovulation in patients with an inadequate response to clomiphene citrate. Fertilsteril. 2001;75:305-9.

Prediction and Prevention of Ovarian Hyperstimulation Syndrome

Kausiki Ray Sarkar

■ INTRODUCTION

Ovarian hyperstimulation syndrome (OHSS) is a potentially serious iatrogenic complication of supraphysiologic ovarian stimulation. Most often it develops in in vitro fertilization (IVF) cycles but can occur in any form of ovarian stimulation, mainly with polycystic ovaries. Though the incidence quoted in different studies varies from 0.2–10%, it may reach up to 20% among high-risk women (Li HW et al, 2014). It is a nightmare for the fertility clinicians, because some forms of OHSS are life threatening. Finnish registry in 2005 concluded incidence of severe OHSS of 1.4% per cycle. Because OHSS is the most serious side effect of COS, clinicians need to be more careful identifying patients who are at risk.

Ovarian hyperstimulation syndrome occurs as a consequence of the cystic enlargement of the ovaries with multiple follicles and a fluid shift from the intravascular to the third space due to increased capillary permeability and ovarian neoangiogenesis. Exact pathophysiology is unknown, but the main culprit is vascular endothelial growth factor (VEGF) which increases the permeability.[1] In response to human chorionic gonadotropin (HCG), VEGF level increases in the system, causing hypovolemia and hyponatremia. Other systemic and local vasoactive substances, like interleukin-6, interleukin1b, angiotensin II, insulin-like growth factor 1, transforming growth factor b, and the renin-angiotensin system are also directly and indirectly involved in the pathogenesis of OHSS symptoms.

There are different predictors or risk factors by which the proneness for OHSS can be determined and reduction of which significantly alter the incidence of OHSS.

1. Demographic factors

    Age and low BMI: According to SART database, largest study with 214, 219 ART cycles, showed many factors which increase the risk, like younger age, black race, ovulation, tubal factor, and unexplained infertility, but age <35 and low BMI are the important ones.[2] It had been seen that more than 60% of affected were below 35 years. Regarding BMI the data is a bit confusing. It is commonly said as low BMI causes increased risk, but at the same time, polycystic ovary syndrome (PCOS) patients, who are commonly overweight, bear more risk.

2. Biochemical markers

Anti müllerian hormone (AMH): AMH levels are nowadays the most important predictor tool for OHSS worldwide. In a comparative study by Ocal et al. in 2011, predictive value of AMH and antral follicle count (AFC) was studied in agonist cycles by comparing 41 cases of OHSS versus 41 non-OHSS. The cutoff value for AMH 3.3 ng/mL has given the highest sensitivity (90%) and specificity (71%). Another study carried out in antagonist cycles with the cutoff of 3.52 ng/mL showed sensitivity 89.5%, and specificity 83.8%. So the cutoff which is being considered as optimum is approx >3.5 ng/mL value, and the higher the value, the higher the risk. One practical thing needs to be mentioned here, that to get a correct value of AMH, the sample must be assessed within 24 hours of collection.

Estradiol (E2): Occurrence of OHSS is almost always accompanied by elevated estradiol level. Now the question is –what will be the cut off for E2 which will be considered detrimental. A study by Asch et al, 1991 found, none of the patients with E2 <3500 pg/mL developed OHSS whereas 1.5% of those having value of 3500–5999 pg/mL and 38% of patients with value of >6000 pg/mL developed OHSS. Another study mentioned that, a rapid increase in E2 levels and serum E2 concentrations >2500 pg/mL was thought to be important predictive factors.[2] Though recent studies have concluded that isolated E2 value is incapable of independently forecasting OHSS and also ESHRE guideline for ovarian stimulation does not recommend the use of E2 for monitoring ovarian response, still for practical take home note, high E2 is always detrimental and to avoid landing up on OHSS either need cycle cancellation or coasting.

3. Ultrasonographic (USG) features

Antral follicle count (AFC) and PCOS patients: AFC has been found to be one of the strongest predictors apart from AMH and its response to stimulation is directly correlated to 'the severity' of OHSS. Though PCO patients act variedly on stimulation, some showing resistance to COH while some with exaggerated response, per se the definition of PCO with high AFC put those patients in high risk category.

4. In Treatment Risk Factors

Response to ovarian stimulation and oocytes retrieved: Various studies have shown that the number of growing follicles is the direct predictors of OHSS. The cut off of growing follicle suggested by Falcone et al, 2012 was 24. Another study by Georg Griesinger et al in 2016 revealed that AUC for the number of follicles ≥11 mm on the day of hCG was 0.728 and the association with moderate to severe OHSS was statistically significant (P <0.0001). For the prediction of moderate to severe OHSS, the optimal threshold was 19 follicles.[3] The sensitivity and specificity were 62.3% and 75.6%, respectively. The percentage of subjects at 'higher risk' that actually experienced moderate to severe OHSS was 6.9% (positive predictive value). Another retrospective analysis, was performed by Tarlatzi et al during a 5-year period (2009–2014) in a single university fertility center, in 2017 revealed the cut off as ≥15. Values are to be noted with caution as all the patients in the above mentioned study were triggered with HCG, not the agonist.

5. Fresh embryo transfer and more number of embryos transferred—Embryo transfer on the stimulation cycles were previously practiced in most of the centers as vitrification was not up to the mark at that period with reversal rate <90%. A study by Mathur et al., in 2000, revealed that Early OHSS was appreciably severe in those cycles which were ending in conception (*P* <0.001), rather than cycles with negative outcome. The same study also mentioned, that the severity was directly proportionate to the number of gestational sacs.

■ PREVENTION POLICIES

1. *Optimization of the stimulation protocol:* In 2016 study within the Engage, Ensure and Trust trials 2585 women were treated with different dosage of either corifollitropin alfa or rFSH and HCG. In total, 2526 women received hCG for oocyte maturation of whom 2433 were assessed for the number of follicles ≥11 mm on day of hCG administration and E2 evaluation. In these women, a total of 136 cases of OHSS were observed: 34 as moderate and 35 as severe. When the dosage of FSH was reduced, a huge change is observed in the occurrence of OHSS. In these trials, the dose of rFSH was reduced in 24%, 22%, and 7% of women, respectively, and the cycle was cancelled in 0.3%, 0% and 0%, respectively, due to risk of OHSS. So optimization of FSH dose is always a key point while stimulating women with high AFC and AMH.

2. *Avoiding HCG trigger:* The fact being HCG causes the stimulated enlarged ovaries to produce the angiogenic molecule VEGF, always cause the flare, whatever be the doses. So apart from decreasing the dose of gonado-tropins, trigger should always be done with GnRH agonist, particularly in high risk patients. Triggering the ovulation using GnRH agonists instead of hCG, first introduced by Itskovitz in 1991 has proven efficacy. Itskovitz-Eldor et al., 2000 had a clinical trial in egg donors using gonadotropin-releasing hormone (GnRH) antagonist protocol and then GnRH agonist to trigger a mid-cycle LH surge, with no cases of OHSS reported.

3. *Freeze all technique:* Cochrane review has illustrated insufficient evidence to support routine cryopreservation by vitrification. According to Cochrane review sequential protocol with freeze all technique does not negate OHSS incidence fully, but 35% reduction occurs in the

incidence. Strengths, weaknesses, opportunities, and threats (SWOT) analysis by Blockeel et al. has thrown light on different aspects of freeze all strategy for prevention of OHSS. It was initially a "rescue" strategy for women at high risk of ovarian hyperstimulation syndrome; however, this approach has been extended to other indications as a scheduled strategy to improve implantation rates (2020 review by Bourdon et al). Dr Paul Devroey and his colleagues in Brussels have put forward a new concept of segmentation approach, where GnRH antagonist protocol, Agonist trigger, cryopreservation of all embryos followed by eSET in a natural or HRT cycle are the mainstay. This protocol is gaining popularity nowadays.

4. *Dopamine agonist therapy and metformin for PCOS:* Recent evidence shows that administration of cabergoline or quinagolide can decrease incidence of OHSS by targeting non-phosphorylation of VEGFR-2.

At the end, sharing some good news with all, that rate of moderate/severe OHSS is definitely falling worldwide. CDC's National ART surveillance system (NASS) shows, OHSS did increase from 2000 to 2006 from 9.96 to 14.4 cases per thousand, but thereafter began a decline to 5.27 per thousand in 2015, with definite fall in severe cases too. From ESHRE database also we are getting the same statistics.[5] So the bottom line is as par a new cohort study from a national US database which confirms COS, with <15 follicles in antagonist cycle with agonist trigger and a freeze-all approach to avoid immediate pregnancy is the pathway towards OHSS free clinic.

REFERENCES

1. Deepika K, Snehal D, Gautham P, Suvarna R, Amit U, Kamini R. Gonadotropin-releasing hormone agonist trigger is a better alternative than human chorionic gonadotropin in PCOS undergoing IVF cycles for an OHSS Free Clinic: A Randomized control trial. J Hum Reprod Sci. 2016;9(3):164-72.
2. Sood A, Mathur R. Prediction of ovarian hyperstimulation syndrome. Fertil Sci Res. 2022;9:5-9.
3. Aboulghar M. Prediction of ovarian hyperstimulation syndrome (OHSS): Oestradiol level has an important role in the prediction of OHSS. Human Reproduction. 2003;18(6):1140-41.
4. Georg Griesinger, Pierre JM Verweij, Davis Gates, Paul Devroey, Keith Gordon, Barbara J. Stegmann, and Basil C. Tarlatzi Prediction of Ovarian Hyperstimulation Syndrome in Patients Treated with Corifollitropin alfa or rFSH in a GnRH Antagonist Protocols. PLoS One. 2016;11(3):e0149615.
5. Rates of OHSS in assisted reproduction continue to fall. ESHRE news, published on July, 2020.

Poor Responders: How to Get the Best Out of the Worst

Asha Baxi, Rajeev Agarwal

INTRODUCTION

Poor response in in vitro fertilization (IVF) treatment was first reported by Garcia et al. in 1983. It is a complex immuno-biochemical process, which is a gray area in IVF treatment. Till date 25% of the patients undergoing ovarian stimulation for IVF, diagnosed as poor responders. In 2011, European society for human reproduction and embryology (ESHRE) came up with the first standardized definition of POR[1] as Bologna criteria.

According to Bologna criteria, poor response in IVF has been defined when at least two of the following three features are present: (i) advanced maternal age (≥40 years) or any other risk factor for poor ovarian response; (ii) a previous POR (less than 3 oocyte retrieved); and (iii) an abnormal ovarian reserve test (AFC lees than 7 or Anti-Müllerian Hormone (AMH) less than 1.1 ng/mL). History of POR after maximal stimulation in the absence of advanced maternal age or abnormal ovarian reserve test (ORT) is also considered as poor response.

Patient oriented strategies encompassing individualized oocyte number (POSEIDON) group has introduced a modified definition of "impaired ovarian response". They have proposed two main categories depending on age, oocyte yield and ovarian reserve – "unexpected" poor responders and "expected" poor responders.

Both the categories are again divided into four groups where group 1 and group 2 consist of "unexpected" poor responders and group 3 and 4 comprises of "expected" poor responders. This classification is based on three parameters: (i) quantitative and qualitative parameters such as age and the expected aneuploidy rate; (ii) ovarian reserve biomarkers (AFC and/or AMH); and (iii) ovarian response—provided a previous stimulation cycle has been performed.[2]

Women in group 1 and 2 are young, with better ORT and have lesser risk of aneuploidy, whereas in group 2 and 4, the risk of embryo aneuploidy is higher due to their age.

47% of all IVF patients are considered as POSEIDON population. More importantly 55% of these belonged to group 4 and 10% in group 3.

PROTOCOLS FOR IN VITRO FERTILIZATION TREATMENT IN POOR RESPONDERS

Pituitary Suppression

Pituitary suppression before stimulation can be done by using estrogen, progestogen, and oral contraceptive pill (OCP), GnRH agonist and antagonist. This suppression is required to achieve synchronized development of adequate number of follicles. However, ESHRE recommendation does not endorse use of estrogen or progesterone due to paucity of strong evidence. No significant difference was seen in ongoing pregnancy rate and live birth rate (LBR) or oocytes yield while using OCP.

Use of Gonadotropins

Regarding Gonadotropins, there is no robust evidence to comment on the efficacy of different types of gonadotropins. There is some evidence that the addition of recombinant human LH (rhLH) to rFSH may have beneficial effects on outcomes in women with POR. This combination results in improved follicular recruitment, and a reduced rate of granulosa cell apoptosis.

In a meta-analysis in 2017, on comparing long agonist protocol with antagonist, there was no difference in LBR, CPR, and oocyte yield.

Ming-Chao Huang in their study concluded that GnRH agonist long protocol was more effective than GnRH antagonist protocol in young patients with diminished ovarian reserve (DOR).

In agonist group injection Leuprolide acetate 0.5 mg daily was commenced from mid luteal phase of their pretreatment cycle. Human Menopausal Gonadotropin (hMG) of 300 IU was started from day 2 or day 3 of menstruation. Same dose of gonadotropin was used in antagonist protocol where antagonist Cetrorelix 0.25 mg daily started on 6th day of hMG stimulation. They found lower LBR in antagonist group, though it was not statistically significant.

In another study, Sunkara et al. compared long agonist protocol with short agonist and antagonist regime. In long agonist protocol where 400 micrograms of GnRH agonist was used as nasal spray once daily for 2 weeks, commenced in the mid-luteal phase. The dose was reduced to 200 micrograms daily with the onset of ovarian stimulation with gonadotropin. For antagonist protocol, dose of 0.25 mg daily was started when the lead follicle reached 14 mm. They concluded that long agonist protocol and antagonist regime was better than short agonist protocol which retrieved less oocytes.

In a prospective RCT, GnRH agonist stop protocol has been used where GnRH agonist was stopped with the onset of menstruation. They found that early cessation of GnRH analogue is associated with significantly higher number of oocyte retrieval.

Stop GnRH analogue in combination with letrozole priming and GnRH antagonist was used in another study which resulted in significantly higher number of follicles >13 mm on the day of hCG administration and higher number of oocytes (Orvieto, 2021). Here, Letrozole 5mg/day was started and continued for five days followed by higher dose of gonadotropins. When the dominant follicle reach 13 mm, antagonist 0.5mg/day was commenced till hCG trigger. This regimen focuses on the POSEIDON Group 4.

Mild and Minimal Stimulation

In Mild and minimal stimulation, lesser dose of gonadotropins are used in GnRH antagonist cycles along with Clomiphene Citrate (CC), or aromatase inhibitors which resulted in similar clinical outcome as compared to classical long protocol with high dose gonadotropins. Here, the dose of clomiphene citrate is 100 mcg/day or aromatase inhibitor 5 mg/day starting from day 2 of menstruation and continued for 5 days followed by human menopausal gonadotropin hMG150 IU subcutaneously.

Dual Stimulation

Dual stimulation, proposed by Kuang et al.[3], is when the ovarian stimulation is done both in follicular and luteal phase. The first stimulation was started with CC 25 mg per day from day 3 until ovulation trigger, combined with aromatase inhibitor (Letrozole) 2.5 mg per day starting on day 3 for 4 days, and hMG 150 IU every other day starting on Day 6 until the ovulation trigger. Second stimulation was started with Letrozole 2.5 mg/day and hMG 225 IU/day from the day of first oocyte retrieval until second ovulation trigger. Final oocyte maturation was induced by GnRH agonist Triptorelin 0.1mg. NSAIDS (Ibuprofen 600 mg) was given for 2 days, starting from the day of ovulation trigger, to prevent premature LH surge. No GnRH antagonist was used for prevention of premature LH surge.

By using dual stimulation at least 1-6 embryos can be created according to this study.

This approach reduces the risk of cycle cancellation, maximized oocyte yield per stimulation and there is an increase in obtaining a single euploid blastocyst from 42.3–65.5% (Valarelli 2018).

Regarding adjuvant therapy, uniform consensus is lacking in use of Growth hormone, testosterone, dehydroepiandrosterone (DHEA), aspirin, and sildenafil.

Natural IVF cycle is not recommended in poor responders.

INDIVIDUALIZATION OF TREATMENT PROTOCOLS FOR POSEIDON GROUP

Management of Group 1 (<35 years, AFC ≥5, AMH ≥1.2 ng/mL)

These patients require higher dose of gonadotropin due to their suboptimal stimulation. Their oocyte yield and Clinical Pregnancy Rate (CPR) is higher in spite of having normal ORT or inadequate response in previous cycle.

Dual stimulation can be considered in this group.

Management of Group 2 (>35 years, AFC ≥5 but with a History of Unexpected Poor Response, AMH = 1.2 ng/mL)

The risk of aneuploidy and decrease in euploid embryos is associated with this POSEIDON group.

Antagonist protocol and long GnRH agonist protocol are preferred to short GnRH agonist protocol in this group. Gonadotropin is used in the range of 150–225 IU daily for stimulation.

Management of Group 3 and 4 (Women with AMH Value <1.2 ng/mL and AFC <5)

Sunkara[4] in their study used long protocol for good synchronization of the follicle to enhance the number of oocytes. Another retrospective study showed higher LBR by using GnRH antagonist Protocol in POSEIDON group.[3] Combination of recombinant LH and Recombinant FSH is superior to hMG with regard to CPR. Dual stimulation is effective in this group with high ongoing pregnancy rate.

Recent advancement in IVF treatment is use of ART calculator which plays an important role in these subset of patients. This calculator measures the number of oocytes required to get at least one euploid blastocyst for transfer. On the basis of age, sperm quality and number of mature metaphase II (M II) oocyte, the calculator can automatically make two types of predictions. It calculates the minimum number of oocyte required for a single euploid blastocyst and the actual number of mature oocyte retrieved. The above predictors helped in creating final logistic regression analysis model.[5]

■ CONCLUSION

Poor ovarian response is still a major challenge for ART clinicians. There has been evolution in definition of poor ovarian response and risk stratification due to the Poseidon classification. It not only helps clinicians to identify the poor responders but also assists to formulate individualized treatment plan to achieve maximum success. The invention of ART Calculator has made it easier to obtain at least one euploid blastocyst for transfer in each patient. Nevertheless, overall outcome of ovarian stimulation and subsequent reproductive outcome of this subset of patients remains suboptimal till date.

■ REFERENCES

1. Ferraretti AP, La Marca A, Fauser BC, Tarlatzis B, Nargund G, Gianaroli L. ESHRE working group on Poor Ovarian Response Definition. ESHRE consensus on the

definition of "poor response" to ovarian stimulation for in vitro fertilization: The Bologna criteria. Hum Reprod. 2011;26(7):1616-24.

2. Esteves SC, Roque M, Bedoschi GM, Conforti A, Humaidan P, Alviggi C. Defining Low Prognosis Patients Undergoing Assisted Reproductive Technology: POSEIDON Criteria-The Why. Front Endocrinol (Lausanne). 2018;17(9):461. doi: 10.3389/fendo.2018.00461. PMID: 30174650; PMCID: PMC6107695.

3. Kuang Y, Chen Q, Hong Q, Luy Q, AiA, Fu Y, Shoham Z. Double stimulation during the follicular and luteal phases of poor responder in IVF/ICSI programmes. Reprod Biomed Online. 2014;29(6):684-91.

4. Sunkara SK, Rittenberg V, Raine-Fenning N, Bhattacharya S, Zamora J, Coomarasamy A. Association between the number of eggs and live birth in IVF treatment: an analysis of 400 135 treatment cycles. Hum Reprod. 2011; 26:1768-74.

5. Esteves S, Carvalho J, Bento F, Santos J. A novel predictive model to estimate the number of mature oocytes required for obtaining at least one euploid blastocyst for transfer in couples undergoing in vitro fertilization/intracytoplasmic sperm injection: the ART calculator. Front Endocrinol. 2019;2019:99.

Endometrial Preparation for Frozen Thaw Embryo Transfer Cycle

Ameet Patki, Khyati Pandya

■ INTRODUCTION

Ovarian stimulation commonly results in more embryos than are necessary for the fresh embryo transfer cycle. Hence the need for cryopreservation and subsequent replacement of frozen thawed embryos (FET). This is an integral part of assisted reproductive technique programs. In recent years, improvements in laboratory conditions and limitations on the number of embryos to be transferred have led to a progressive increase in FET cycles. This contributes to around 25% of all births achieved by ART[1]. However, the best protocol for endometrial preparation in these cycles is still a matter of debate.

Cryopreservation and subsequent FET prevents embryo waste and increases the probability of pregnancy in a single stimulated cycle. Protocols applied in FET cycles aim for endometrial preparation only and are therefore simpler than complicated protocols of stimulation. Frozen embryo transfer increases the cumulative pregnancy rate and decreases the cost; it is easy to perform and can be finished in a shorter time duration when compared to repetitive fresh embryo transfers[2].

Embryo implantation represents the most critical step of the reproductive process in many species. It consists of a unique biological phenomenon, by which the blastocyst becomes intimately connected to the maternal endometrial surface to form the placenta that will provide an interface between the growing fetus and the maternal circulation. Successful implantation requires a receptive endometrium, a normal and functional embryo at the blastocyst developmental stage and a synchronized dialogue between maternal and embryonic tissues. The process of implantation may be classified into three stages: apposition, adhesion and invasion. During blastocyst apposition, trophoblast cells adhere to the receptive endometrial epithelium. The blastocyst will subsequently anchor to the endometrial basal lamina and stromal extracellular matrix (ECM). At this point, the achieved embryo–endometrial linkage can no longer be dislocated by uterine flushing. This is followed by the invasive blastocyst penetration through the luminal epithelium.

It is vital that a frozen – thawed embryo is replaced during the window of endometrial receptivity and that there is synchronization between embryo and endometrial development. There have been a number of different protocols developed to achieve this; namely-

- Replacement during a natural ovulatory cycle.
- Hormone (estrogen and progesterone) replacement cycles (with or without prior downregulation).
- Ovulation induction cycles.

There is growing evidence that endometrial receptivity may be negatively affected by ovarian stimulation. Recent studies have suggested that there may be an advantage to freezing all blastocysts in the fresh cycle and replacing them in a natural or downregulated cycle.

■ NATURAL FROZEN EMBRYO TRANSFER CYCLE

In natural frozen embryo transfer cycles, the easiest is the endocrinological preparation of the endometrium during the natural cycle using the patient's own follicular sex steroids. In this method the timing for embryo transfer (ET) is determined by either determining the spontaneous luteinizing hormone (LH) surge or by the administration of exogenous hCG to start luteinization. Success of the natural cycle depends on the accurate determination of the ovulation time and the precise estimation of endometrial receptivity to detect the LH surge. The major advantage of replacement of embryos in a woman's natural ovulatory cycle is that no medication is required. However, there will be significant proportion of women in whom this approach will not be suitable like women with anovulatory PCOS.

Thawing and transfer procedures have to be performed during this receptive period. In FET cycles performed during a natural cycle, urine or blood LH level is regularly analyzed and followed up. Ovulation is estimated to occur 36 to 40 hours after the presence of the blood LH surge. Urine LH increases 21 hours after the detection of the blood LH surge, and this fact has to be taken into consideration when interpreting the increase in urine LH.

A problem in determining the time of the spontaneous LH surge is the variability of this increase, both among cycles and patients. At least one measurement, and preferably two measurements, has to be performed daily in order to accurately determine the LH surge. The threshold values of urine LH kits are highly variable, corresponding to an approximately 30% risk of a false-negative result; additionally patients state that it is hard to interpret the test results.

Some clinics advocate the use of HCG to trigger ovulation and aid in the timing of embryo replacement. A small RCT has shown that the use of an HCG trigger decreases the monitoring visits required in the natural cycle FET with no difference in the pregnancy outcome. In natural or modified natural cycles, the embryo transfer is performed three to five days after ovulation, depending on when the embryos were frozen.

Ovulation may occur unexpectedly while planning a natural cycle, which can lead to difficulties in adjusting the time of thawing and transferring the embryos. When an unexpected early ovulation occurs, the cycle is generally cancelled.

HORMONE REPLACEMENT CYCLE

Another frequently used method for endometrium preparation is with the exogenous administration of estrogen and progesterone (with or without a gonadotrophin-releasing-hormone (GnRH) agonist), also called the artificial cycle, and is frequently used as an alternative for the natural cycle. Rates of clinical pregnancy and chemical pregnancy were shown not to differ in artificial cycles with regard to the administration of a GnRH agonist.[5]

One possible advantage of medicated FET is that it allows flexibility as to the timing of embryo transfer that may suit both the patient and the clinic. A number of different protocols exist for the artificial cycles.

First, ovarian downregulation can be achieved by the use of a GnRH agonist, after which sequential estrogen with subsequent addition of progesterone is used.

Estrogens can be administered by various routes, i.e., oral, patches or intramuscular injections. No route has shown to have any clear advantages over others. However amongst the compounds 17β estradiol had advantages over estradiol valerate being more physiological and less side effects.

Similarly progestogens can also be administered by oral, vaginal or intramuscular routes. No route has shown to have any clear advantages over others. However oral dydrogesterone has shown to be significantly better in some studies.[6] Blastocyst transfer occurs after 5 days of progesterone administration.

In order to mimic the endocrine conditions of the endometrium of a normal cycle in an artificial cycle, estrogen and progesterone are administered consecutively. Estrogen administration is started at the beginning of the cycle, causing endometrial development while suppressing dominant follicle development ideally as early as 2nd day of menses. Estrogen administration is continued until the endometrium reaches a thickness of 8 mm, and progesterone is then combined to initiate the secretory changes thereby to mimic the physiologic mid-cycle estrogen–progesterone transition.

In artificial preparation, the time for thawing and transferring the embryos is planned according to the commencement of progesterone support. The exogenous administration of estrogen and progesterone does not always guarantee the complete suppression of the pituitary gland; in other words, a dominant follicle may develop. The developing follicle may also undergo spontaneous luteinization, which leads to the early exposure of the endometrium to progesterone, and thus incorrect calculations for thawing and transfer times. In such cases GnRH agonists can be added to the treatment protocols in order to downregulate the pituitary, thus preventing follicular development.

In the meta-analysis of studies comparing estrogen and progesterone with and without a GnRH analogue, there was no significant difference in the cycle cancellation, endometrial thickness, pregnancy rates or miscarriage rate.

STIMULATED REGIMES FOR FROZEN EMBRYO TRANSFER CYCLE

An alternative approach to endometrial preparation for the frozen embryo transfer cycle is to use low dose ovarian stimulation. One RTC of 199 women compared the use of 150 IU FSH on day 6, 8 and 10 of the menstrual cycle to estrogen and progesterone endometrial preparation (with no prior downregulation). No differences were identified in the implantation or pregnancy rate, cancellation rate, or endometrial thickness.[7] Clomiphene citrate has also been used for stimulation but the only RTC using this intervention showed no benefit over estrogen and progesterone, used with or without a GnRH analogue.[8] Ovulation induction cycles have no benefits in terms of pregnancy rate. In addition, they require increased monitoring, are relatively expensive, and do not have the advantage of flexibility with regards to the timing of the embryo transfer.

ERA (ENDOMETRIAL RECEPTIVITY ARRAY)

This is a genetic test that diagnoses the state of endometrial receptivity in the window of implantation in women. This molecular diagnostic tool is used to analyze the expression level of 238 genes related to the status of endometrial receptivity. An in house designed computational predictor analyses the data obtained, classifying the endometrium as receptive or non- receptive.[9]

The use of this test in patients with recurrent implantation has shown that the window of implantation is displaced in a quarter of these patients and use of a personalized embryo transfer on the day designated by ERA improves reproductive performance.

Endometrial receptivity now appears to be the bottleneck of the reproductive process. Basic and clinical research will help to better understand the events of uterine preparation for embryo implantation. Novel in vivo approaches, including additives to the embryo culture or intrauterine flushing with putative adhesion promoting factors, could potentially increase implantation rates especially in repeated implantation failure. Endometrial biopsy samples can be used to identify molecules associated with uterine receptivity to obtain a better insight into human implantation. In addition, development of functional in vitro systems to study embryo-uterine interactions will better define the interactions existing between the molecules involved in this process. Up to date, only a few modalities have been employed to treat failures of conception, despite the repeated transfer of apparently good quality embryos. The methods reported in the literature including medium supplementation by hyaluronic acid, administration of LIF, progesterone, drugs like NSAIDs and heparin. With the exception of luteal phase support by progesterone administration, none of the treatments cited above was shown to be efficient in increasing implantation or pregnancy rates. Future research, therefore, must be directed towards deciphering the functional, rather than the morphological characteristics of endometrial receptivity. The knowledge acquired will assist investigators in the development of specific molecular markers of endometrial receptivity.

Embryo implantation is the result of a well-orchestrated sequence of events including cellular adhesion, invasion and immune regulatory mechanisms, some of which are controlled through genetic processes by the ovarian hormones.

■ REFERENCES

1. Nygren KG, Sullivan E, Zegers-Hochschild F, et al. International committee for monitoring assisted reproductive technology (ICMART) world report: assisted reproductive technology 2003. Fertil Steril. 2011;95:2209-22; 22e1-17.

2. Shapiro BS, Daneshmand ST, Garner FC, Aguirre M, Hudson C, Thomas S. Evidence of impaired endometrial receptivity after ovarian stimulation for in vitro fertilization: a prospective randomized trial comparing fresh and frozen-thawed embryo transfer in normal responders. Fertil Steril. 2004;96(2):344-8.

3. Wright KP, Guibert J, Weitzen S, Davy C, Fauque P, Olivennes F. Artificial versus stimulated cycles for endometrial preparation prior to frozen–thawed embryo transfer. Reprod Biomed Online. 2006;13:321-5.

4. Imbar T, Hurwitz A. Synchronization between endometrial and embryonic age is not absolutely crucial for implantation. Fertil Steril. 2004;82:472-4.

5. El-Toukhy T, Coomarasamy A, Khairy M, Sunkara K, Seed P, Khalaf Y, et al. The relationship between endometrial thickness and outcome of medicated frozen embryo replacement cycles. Fertil Steril. 2008;89:832-9.

6. Patki AS, Pawar V. Modulating Fertility Outcome in Assisted Reproductive Technologies by The Use of Dydrogesterone. Gynaecological Endocrinology. 2007;23(S1):1-5.

7. Wright KP, Guibert J, Weitzen S, et al. Artificial versus stimulated cycles for endometrial preparation prior to frozen thawed embryo transfer. Reprod Biomed Online. 2006;13:321-5.

8. Loh SKE, Ganesan G, Leong NK. Clomid versus hormone endometrial preparation in FET cycles. Abstract book of the 17th world congress in fertility and sterility (IFFS). Melbourne, Australia. 2001;3:25-30.

9. Maria Ruiz-Alonso, David Blesa, Patricia Díaz-Gimeno, Eva Gómez, Manuel Fernández-Sánchez, Francisco Carranza, Joan Carrera, Felip Vilella, Antonio Pellicer, Carlos Simón, The endometrial receptivity array for diagnosis and personalized embryo transfer as a treatment for patients with repeated implantation failure, Fertility and Sterility. 2013;100(3):818-24.

Elective Single Embryo Transfer

Hrishikesh D Pai, Manisha T Kundnani, Arnav Pai

■ INTRODUCTION

In vitro fertilization (IVF) has proven to be a boon for many infertile couples in the past few decades. On one hand where it has given hopes to many, it has also introduced many risks. One of the major complications in IVF since its inception has been multiple gestation and its associated perinatal and maternal complications. Controlled ovarian stimulation is the integral part of all IVF programs which often results in multiple good grade embryos available for transfer. It is a common practice in almost all clinics to transfer more than one embryo in a cycle to enhance the success rates. However, this practice of transferring more than one embryo also results in higher incidences of iatrogenic twins and high orders multiple gestations, which causes significant maternal and perinatal morbidity.

While strict transfer policies have eliminated the risk of high order multiples, the incidence of twin pregnancy is still unchanged. Selective fetal reduction is often being used to reduce these multiple gestations, but the procedure is invasive and is associated with its own cons. Elective single embryo transfer and cryopreservation of spare embryos is a good strategy to avoid multiple and twin pregnancies in IVF and its allied complications. Traditionally embryos have been selected based on morphology, but morphological selection is not always predictive of implantation potential. PGT, time lapse imaging, artificial intelligence, and metabolomics are additional tools which may/can help in better selection of a euploid embryo with highest implantation potential. Proper patient selection for elective single embryo transfer (eSET), good patient counselling and selection of best embryo for implantation are important factors in adopting this policy.

■ ELECTIVE SINGLE EMBRYO TRANSFER

Elective single embryo transfer is defined as the intentional transfer of a single embryo (cleavage stage or blastocyst stage), despite the availability of more than one good grade embryos. This is different from obligatory or non-elective SET where only one embryo is available for transfer.

The notion behind this practice is to eliminate the risk of twins and higher order multiple pregnancies, and the associated maternal, perinatal, and neonatal complication akin with these high orders assisted reproductive technology (ART) conceptions.

Maternal and Perinatal Complications with Multiple Pregnancies

Though the advances in the neonatal care have significantly reduced the neonatal morbidity and mortality, multiple gestation still carry a substantial risk to the mother and the child. Multiple pregnancies carry a higher risk of pregnancy induced hypertension, gestational diabetes, preterm delivery, low birth weight, higher incidence of birth defects and neurological problems like cerebral palsy.

Not only multiple pregnancy cause significant health issues, it also leads to tremendous increase in the cost of healthcare. It has been estimated that maternal and infant healthcare cost of twin pregnancies is 3–5 times higher, and that of triplet pregnancy is approximately 20 times higher compared to a singleton pregnancy. Besides the health risks, it has been observed that the increased emotional, physical and financial stress leads to a higher incidence of depression and anxiety disorders in these parents. A higher incidence of postpartum depression is also reported in women rearing multiples compared to singleton babies. E-SET can completely eliminate these risks associated with higher order gestations.

◼ SINGLE vs. DOUBLE EMBRYO TRANSFER

Success Rates

It has been observed that the live birth rate with only single cycle with SET is lower to DET (double embryo transfer) by almost 7%. DET however is associated with substantially higher incidence of multiple gestations. In a prospective randomized study conducted by Lopez Regalado et al, in women less than 38 years and with good prognosis, it was observed that cumulative live birth rates after eSET followed by a transfer of single frozen embryo are similar to those seen with single DET (45% vs. 42%), with a zero incidence of multiple gestations in SET compared to 28% in DET.[1] Similar findings were then observed by multiple other researchers suggesting SET plus subsequent frozen eSET is as effectual as DET.[2-4] Shujuan et al., recently conducted a meta-analysis comparing the benefits and risks of SET vs. DET. The authors concluded that in women <40 years, if any good quality embryo is available, SET should be done. If no good quality embryos are available, DET can be preferred. For women >40 years, evidence is limited to recommend an appropriate number of embryo to be transferred.[5]

TABLE 1: Barriers to elective single embryo transfer (eSET).

- Lower perceived success rates with SET
- Lack of knowledge about risks associated with multiple gestations
- Extra costs of freezing and thawing
- High costs of multiple IVF cycles
- Lack of medical insurance for fertility treatments
- Desire for siblings

BARRIERS TO ELECTIVE SINGLE EMBRYO TRANSFER (TABLE 1)

Single embryo transfer can completely eliminate the risks associated with the multiple pregnancies and can help achieve the ultimate goal of infertility treatment, i.e. single healthy baby. But still this practice has not gained widespread use. Various factors impede the widespread adoption of this policy. Perceived lower success rates with SET compared with double or multiple embryo transfer is an important factor impeding the uptake of eSET. Infertility patients want to maximize the chances of pregnancy and their desire to become pregnant often outweighs the concerns associated with multiple gestations and the problems associated with rearing multiple children simultaneously.

Lack of patient awareness about the risk associated with multiple pregnancies; and the desire to reduce the emotional, physical and financial stress of multiple IVF cycles are the other factors limiting the use of eSET. In addition, many couples often express the desire for siblings and are thus more willing to accept the risk of multiple pregnancies. It has been observed that women with advanced age and longer duration of infertility (>2 years) are more likely to desire for multiple births.

High costs of multiple IVF cycles and limited insurance coverage are additional challenges for adopting eSET.

Patient education and counselling, specifically explaining them about the cumulative success rates of SET and frozen embryo transfers, and also the risks and additional costs associated with multiple pregnancies can help them make a decision in favor of SET. Insurance coverage for infertility treatment will take away the additional financial burden of freezing and thawing and can thus help in promoting SET. Enhanced embryo selection techniques can help in better selection of embryo for eSET and can help to empower patients to choose eSET while maintaining high success rates.

Candidates for Elective Single Embryo Transfer

In spite of the proven benefits of eSET, there has been a significant challenge in selecting the appropriate candidate for eSET and implementing an effective eSET protocol. As female age is one of the strongest predictors of IVF success, it is the crucial decisive factor in deciding patients for eSET. Other factors

TABLE 2: ASRM or SART recommended criteria for elective single embryo transfer (eSET).[6]

- Women aged <35years
- Women aged 35-40 years should also consider eSET if they have top quality blastocyst stage embryos available for transfer
- More than one top quality embryo available for transfer-blastocyst stage embryos are preferred
- First or second IVF cycle
- Previously successful IVF cycle
- Recipients of embryos from donated eggs

like the embryo quality and previous IVF attempts also play a crucial role in selecting the patients who would benefit maximum by eSET.

A new term mSET (*medical* SET) is recently introduced and is reserved for women with total or relative contraindication to multifetal gestation because of known medical conditions. These should be informed about the risks of multiple gestations and elective SET should be mandatory in such women.

Absolute contraindications for multiple gestations:

- Congenital uterine Müllerian anomaly, associated with a high risk for preterm birth.
- History of ruptured uterus.
- Cervical incompetence.
- Turner syndrome.
- Severe systemic disease.
- Severe psychiatric disease.
- Early multiple pregnancy loss.
- Insulin-dependent diabetes.

EMBRYO SELECTION FOR ELECTIVE SINGLE EMBRYO TRANSFER

It is prudent to select embryo with the highest implantation potential for eSET so as to have the maximum chance of implantation and live birth. Various techniques allow for better selection of embryos including blastocyst culture, PGT, time lapse, artificial intelligence and metabolomics.

Blastocyst Culture

Elective single blastocyst transfer is found to have superior success rates compared to single cleavage stage (Day 2 or day 3) embryo transfer.[7,8] Further it has been observed that good grade blastocysts as classified by the SART grading system (based on morphology, expansion and overall quality), have better success rates compared to low grade blastocysts.[9] Also, transferring one good grade blastocyst had similar live birth rates compared to transfer of two blastocysts, with significantly reduced multiple birth rates.[10,11]

Role of Preimplantation Genetic Testing in Selecting Embryo for Elective Single Embryo Transfer

Conventionally embryos have been selected based on morphological grading systems. However, it has been observed that morphological selection of embryos is not 100% accurate and approximately 20% of days 5 embryos transferred based on morphological selection alone may be aneuploid.[12] Aneuploidy is the major cause of implantation failure and miscarriages in ART cycles.[13] PGT-A along with comprehensive chromosome screening allows to select euploid embryos and thus can be a can be a useful tool in embryo selection for eSET. Trophectoderm biopsy at blastocyst stage is currently the preferred method for screening.

A prospective randomized study by Scott et al. observed that 96% of aneuploid embryos fail to implant compared to 41% of euploid embryos.[14] In a randomized trial conducted by Forman et al, which included 175 women less than 43 years of age, it was observed that transfer of one euploid embryo results in similar pregnancy rates compared to transfer of two unscreened embryos (69% after euploid eSET compared to 72% after untested DET, p value = 0.6).[15] The incidence of twin pregnancies, preterm deliveries and NICU admissions was significantly lesser in the euploid eSET group. Schoolcraft et al observed that use of CCS can improve eSET success rates in women with advanced maternal age (>35 years).[13] In another study conducted by Gonzalez et al it was observed that euploid blastocysts implant irrespective of their morphology after NGS-(PGT-A) testing in women with advanced age.[16]

However, in spite of various studies proving the benefit of PGS in embryo selection, the technology has not gained widespread use. The additional costs of the procedure, the need for cryopreservation of all embryos and the fact that euploidy does not guarantee pregnancy and successful live birth are the factors limiting its use.

A newer technology called non-invasive chromosome screening (NICS) uses spent culture media to isolate cell free embryonic DNA which is then tested for aneuplodies. The advantage of this technique over conventional PGT is that it is totally non-invasive and does not disturb the growth of the embryo.

Time Lapse Monitoring for Selection of Embryo for Elective Single Embryo Transfer

Traditionally, embryos have been assessed by direct observation under the inverted microscope. Though this method is simple, it is subject to interobserver variability and it provides information of the embryo only at the time of assessment. Time lapse technology is a new milestone in the field of assisted reproduction as it allows for continuous non-invasive observation of embryos. It allows monitoring the embryos without disturbing the culture conditions. The continuous monitoring and the large number of pictures available provide thorough information about the embryo development. It also enables observation of specific developmental events such as multinucleation, direct division (division from one to three cells) and cell fusion. Observing these events is crucial, as they are associated with a low implantation potential.[17] The embryos can thus be selected based on morphological, dynamic and morphokinetic criteria using some predictive programs and algorithms.[18]

An association between embryo aneuploidy and time lapse markers has also been assessed in various studies. It has been observed that euploid embryos follow tight kinetic parameters whereas aneuploid embryos have an unpredictable development outside the optimal range and show a higher degree of fragmentation.

A number of studies have compared outcomes after embryo selection by morphokinetic vs. morphological assessment. Though some researchers found increased success and live birth rates using time lapse, many other did not find any improved outcomes using this technology.[19,20]

Though the concept of time lapse monitoring sounds promising, more prospective studies are needed to prove its efficacy and safety before this can be applied in routine clinical use.[21]

Artificial Intelligence (AI) for Embryo Selection

Both direct visualization and time lapse methods of embryo selection grade embryos based on their ability to reach particular stages of development in timely manner. However, these morphological grading systems remain limited in their ability to predict live birth. Artificial intelligence using routinely generated images or time lapse videos can help to grade embryos more accurately and objectively and can thus help in better embryo selection for e-SET. AI can also have a role in analyzing data from non-invasive metabolomics and secretory profiles from embryo culture media. Though, many studies have shown that AI can help in improving the accuracy of manual grading and predicting development to blastocyst, its usefulness in increasing the LBR is yet to be demonstrated.[22,23]

Metabolomics for Embryo Selection

Metabolomics in ART refers to metabolite product found in specific biological material or media. They are a group of small non-proteinaceous compounds including metabolic intermediates, adenosine triphosphate, hormones or metabolites. They are more informative than genomics, transcriptomics or proteomics as they represent the final product of cell regulatory system and so are closer to the functional phenotype. Metabolomics profiling of embryo is done using spent culture media. Though the technique has helped in better understanding of nutritional environment of oocytes and embryos, it is yet to be proved beneficial for improving ongoing pregnancy and live birth rates.[24]

CONCLUSION

The ultimate goal of infertility treatment is a single healthy baby. Multiple pregnancies are one of the major complications of IVF and there is a global recognition of the need to reduce the incidence of same. eSET is an effective method to reduce multiple gestations following IVF. However, multiple factors like lower perceived success rates with SET; financial, emotional and physical burden of multiple IVF cycles; patients desire for twins and lack of awareness about risks associated with multiple gestations act as barriers in adoption of this technique. Personalized counselling, expanding insurance coverage for IVF, better tools to predict IVF success and technologies to select high quality embryos with best implantation potential would facilitate wider use of eSET. Patient age, previous treatment history and quality of embryos can help select the optimal patients for eSET. Though, technical advances like preimplantation genetic assessment, time lapse monitoring and artificial intelligence have been shown to improve the embryo selection, at present, there is insufficient evidence to recommend the routine use of these new techniques.

REFERENCES

1. Lopez Regalado ML, Clavero A, Gonzalvo MC, et al. Randomised clinical trial comparing elective single embryo transfer followed by single embryo cryotransfer versus double embryo transfer. Eur J Obstet Gynecol Reprod Biol. 2014;178:192-8.
2. Clua E, Tur R, Coroleu B, et al. Is it justified to transfer two embryos in oocyte donation? A pilot randomized clinical trial. Reprod Biomed Online. 2015; 31(2):154-61.
3. Thurin A, Hausken J, HIllensjo T, et al. Elective single embryo transfer vs. double embryo transfer in in vitro fertilization. N Engl J Med. 2004;351:2392-402.
4. Criniti A, Thyer A, Chow G, et al. Elective single blastocyst transfer reduces twin rates without compromising pregnancy rates. Fertil Steril. 2005;84:1613-9.
5. Ma S, Peng Y, Gong F, et al. Comparison of benefits and risks of single embryo transfer versus double embryo transfer: a systematic review and meta-analysis. Reprod Biol Endocrinol. 2022:20-20.
6. American Society for Reproductive Medicine. Elective single embryo transfer. Fertil Steril. 2012;97(4):835-42.
7. Marek D, Langley M, Gardner DK, et al. Introduction of blastocyst culture and transfer for all patients in an in vitro fertilization program. Fertil Steril. 1999;72:1035-40.
8. Papanikolaou EG, Camus M, Kolibianakis EM, et al. In vitro fertilization with single blastocyst stage versus single cleavage stage embryos. N Engl J Med. 2006;354:1139-46.

9. Heitmann RJ, Hill MJ, Richter KS, et al. The simplified SART embryo scoring system is highly correlated to implantation and live birth in single blastocyst transfers. J Assist Reprod Genet. 2013;30:563-7.

10. Gardner DK, Surrey E, Minjarez D, et al. Single blastocyst transfer: a prospective randomized trial. Fertil Steril. 2004;81:551-5.

11. Styer AK, Wright DL, Wolkovich AM, et al. Single blastocyst transfer reduces twin gestation without affecting pregnancy outcome. Fertil Steril. 2008;89:1702-8.

12. Forman EJ, Upham KM, Cheng M, et al. Comprehensive chromosome screening alters traditional morphology based embryo selection: a prospective study of 100 consecutive cycles of planned fresh euploid blastocyst transfer. Fertil Steril. 2013;100:718-24.

13. Schoolcraft WB, Katz-Jaffe MG. Comprehensive chromosome screening of trophoectoderm with vitrification facilitates elective single embryo transfer for infertile women with advanced maternal age. Fertil Steril. 2013;100:615-9.

14. Scott RT Jr, Ferry K, Su J, et al. Comprehensive chromosome screening is highly predictive of the reproductive potential of human embryos: a prospective blinded non selection study. Fertile Steril. 2012;97:870-5.

15. Forman EJ, Hong KH, Franasiak JM, et al. Obstetrical and neonatal outcomes from the BEST trial.: single embryo transfers with aneuploidy screening improves outcomes after in vitro fertilisation without compromising delivery rates. Am J Obstet Gynecol. 2014;10:157.

16. C Gonzalez VX, Odia RE, Naja R, et al. Euploid blastocysts implant irrespective of their morphology after NGS-(PGT-A) testing in advanced maternal age patients. J assist Reprod Genet. 2019;36:1623-9.

17. Barrie A, Homburg R, McDowell, et al. Preliminary investigation of the prevalence and implantation potential of abnormal embryonic phenotypes assessed using time-lapse imaging. Reprod Biomed Online. 2017;34:455-62.

18. Kirkegaard K, Ahlström A, Ingerslev HJ, Hardarson T. Choosing the best embryo by time lapse versus standard morphology. Fertil Steril. 2015;103:323-32.

19. Adamson GD, Abusief ME, Palao L, et al. Improved implantation rates of day 3 embryo transfers with the use of an automated time-lapse–enabled test to aid in embryo selection. Fertil Steril. 2016;105:369-75.

20. Goodman LR, Goldberg J, Falcone T, et al. Does the addition of time-lapse morphokinetics in the selection of embryos for transfer improve pregnancy rates? A randomized controlled trial. Fertil Steril. 2016;105:275-85.

21. Armstrong S, Bhide P, Jordan V, et al. Time-lapse systems for embryo incubation and assessment in assisted reproduction. Cochrane Database Syst Rev. 2019;5: CD011320.

22. Ver Mileya M, Hall JMM, Diakiw SM, et al. Development of an artificial intelligence based assessment model for prediction of embryo viability using static images captured by optical light microscopy during IVF. Hum Reprod. 2020;35:770-84.

23. Chavez Badiola A, Flores-Saifee Farias A, Mendizabal-Ruiz G, et al. Predicting pregnancy test results after embryo transfer by image feature extraction and analysis using machine learning. Scientific reports. 2020;10:4394.

24. Siristatidis CS, Sertedaki E, Vaidakis D, et al. Metabolomics for improving pregnancy outcomes in women undergoing assisted reproductive technologies. Cochrane Database Syst Rev. 2017;23:CD011872.

Pregnancy after ART— Does the Management Differ?

Jaideep Malhotra, Shiuli Mukherjee

INTRODUCTION

Assisted reproductive technology (ART) now accounts for nearly 1.6% of all infants and 18.3% of all multiple-birth infants and nearly 20–25% of total pregnancies in a year. Over the past decades, the use of assisted reproductive technology (ART) has increased dramatically worldwide and has made pregnancy possible for many infertile couples. Although most of these pregnancies are uncomplicated, IVF is occasionally associated with several adverse maternal and perinatal outcomes. Namely multiple gestation, preterm labor, low birth weight baby, IUGR, placental abnormalities and maternal hypertension, PET, GDM and subsequently increasing maternal morbidity and perinatal mortality.[1,2]

PREPREGNANCY WORK-UP

A thorough check up and pre-ART evaluation of mother even with genetic evaluation are needed before taking up the patients for IVF.[3] Even for more common medical disorders (such as diabetes, hypertension, epilepsy, or obesity), optimization of weight, maternal medical status, treatment regimen, and other aspects of care may have salutary effects on becoming pregnant and pregnancy outcomes. Therefore, prepregnancy assessment of pregnancy-related risks and counseling regarding risk reduction strategies should be a key element of care before the initiation of ART or any infertility treatment.

STRATEGIES FOR LIMITING THE RISK OF MULTIPLE GESTATIONS

Multiple gestation increases both maternal and fetal complications. While preeclampsia is 6% in singleton pregnancy but 10–12% in twin, gestational diabetes is 3% in singleton pregnancy and 5–8% in twin. Preterm labor <37 weeks is 2% in single fetus but 8%in twin and 92% in triplet gestation. Small for gestational age (<2500 gm) is found in 6.2 % of single fetus gestation whereas it reaches as high as 93.2% in triplet. Around 37.5% of triplet twin is associated with <1.5kg.[3] So *Elective single embryo transfer (eSET)* has been proposed as the most direct way to limit the risk of multiple gestations. *Multifetal pregnancy reduction(MFR)* is other alternative to decreases the risk of preterm delivery in quadruplets or triplets reduced to twins or to singletons. Termination of one or more fetuses decreases the risk of preterm delivery, although the decrease should be balanced against a procedure-associated risk of miscarriage (approximately 4–5%).[2,3]

Placental abnormalities: The risk of placenta previa may be increased in pregnancies conceived by ART which may be as high as six-fold higher compared with naturally conceived pregnancies. There is also a suggestion that FETs are associated with decreased risk of placenta previa and abruptio placentae, suggesting that the endometrial environment at the time of implantation plays a role in the pathogenesis of these complications.

Preeclampsia: A small increase in the risk of pre-eclampsia has been reported in women undergoing ART in their second and third trimester with more than double the risk in ART via oocyte donation (OD) when compared to other methods of ART and more than a four-fold increased risk compared with natural conception.

■ EARLY PREGNANCY LOSS AND ECTOPIC PREGNANCY

In pregnancies conceived by IVF, it has been found that the spontaneous loss of at least one gestation occurred in approximately 25% of singleton pregnancies, 35% of twin pregnancies, and 55% of triplet pregnancies whereas the rate of second trimester loss does not appear to be impacted by ART. The incidence of ectopic pregnancy has been estimated at 0.7% which could vary according to the type of procedure (higher with zygote intrafallopian transfer or ZIFT) and tubal factor infertility. Heterotopic pregnancy is far more common in ART than spontaneous conceptions (1/100 versus 1/30,000).[3]

■ NEONATAL OUTCOMES

Low Birth Weight

It appears that frozen embryo transfers (FETs) are associated with a decrease in small for gestational age (SGA) and LBW births, as well as with preterm births which could possibly be explained by the more natural endometrial preparation prior to FET allowing for more natural placentation than that which occurs in stimulated cycles.[4]

Congenital Anomalies

The higher risk of congenital anomalies in ART pregnancies may be related to infertility itself or to factors related to ART procedures or both where vanishing twins may also play a role. However, the absolute risk of having a child with congenital anomalies is low.[4]

Chromosomal and Genetic Abnormalities

Karyotypic abnormalities (including mosaicism) have not been found to be higher in pregnancies conceived by IVF and prenatal diagnosis is not typically offered for this indication alone. Subfertile men (and women) are more likely to have chromosomal anomalies (e.g., aneuploidies, structural abnormalities, gene mutations, microdeletions) which may either contribute to their subfertility and may be passed to their fetus. Preimplantation genetic screening can be offered for screening those at specific risk for an inherited disease is supported.[4]

Imprinting Disorders

Imprinting abnormalities occur during DNA mutations of an imprinted gene which occur predominantly during meiosis, typically with alterations of methylations. The rarity of this entity makes it difficult to attribute the cause to ART procedure or subfertility itself or a combination of factors.[4]

■ TO SCREEN OR NOT?

Genetic alterations in methylation, epigenetics, and imprinting have been reported in ART pregnancies that could result in disorders such as Beckwith–Wiedemann and Angelman syndromes. However, no specific pattern of anomalies or disorders has been identified for which targeted screening or evaluation can be endorsed.[5] More importantly, patient's medical history is of paramount importance in identifying patient-specific risks that may indicate need for specific studies or other fetal evaluation during pregnancy.

■ LONG TERM PEDIATRIC OUTCOMES

1. *Nurodevelopmental delay:* There is conflicting results about any increase in adverse neurodevelopmental outcomes due to ART specific interventions or multifetal gestation related prematurity. No differences were detected in a study comparing 253 ART-conceived adolescents (born between 1982 and 1993) with case-matched controls in terms of general health, mental health, or cognitive ability upon review of military preinduction screening records (performed at ages 16 to 17 years).
2. *Risk of future malignancy:* The overall absolute risk is still higher than the general population, however association does not establish causality.
3. *Cardiovascular changes:* Few case reports describing vascular changes like carotid media thickness in children conceived by ART open an area of interest to evaluate the association between ART and cardiovascular changes considering other confounders like fetal growth restriction and prematurity.[5]

FROM EGG TO BABY: WHAT EXTRA CARE DOES ASSISTED REPRODUCTIVE TECHNOLOGY PREGNANCIES NEED?

1. One of the main differences of care for women becoming pregnant using ART to spontaneous pregnancy was for those who became pregnant with IVF-ICSI, because of a higher risk of birth defects and prenatal screening is recommended.
2. Multifetal pregnancies should be avoided, and if they occur, the option of selective reduction should be discussed, including the emotions associated with this and the possibility of loss of the entire pregnancy
3. Counseling prior to treatment, during treatment and during pregnancy forms an integral component of managing ART pregnancies which must include the risks associated with treatment (e.g. multi-fetal pregnancies), risks during pregnancy (e.g., preeclampsia), higher risk deliveries (e.g., postpartum hemorrhage), and risk to the baby (e.g., low birth weight, preterm delivery)
4. *Psychosocial counselling:* ESHRE defines this as the care that enables couples, their families and their health care providers to optimize infertility care and manage the psychological and social implications of infertility and its treatment as most patients experience emotional distress during treatment. ESHRE 2015 guidelines are so far the only guidelines dealing with the psychosocial stress of ART on a time and need axis as depicted in **Figure 1**.

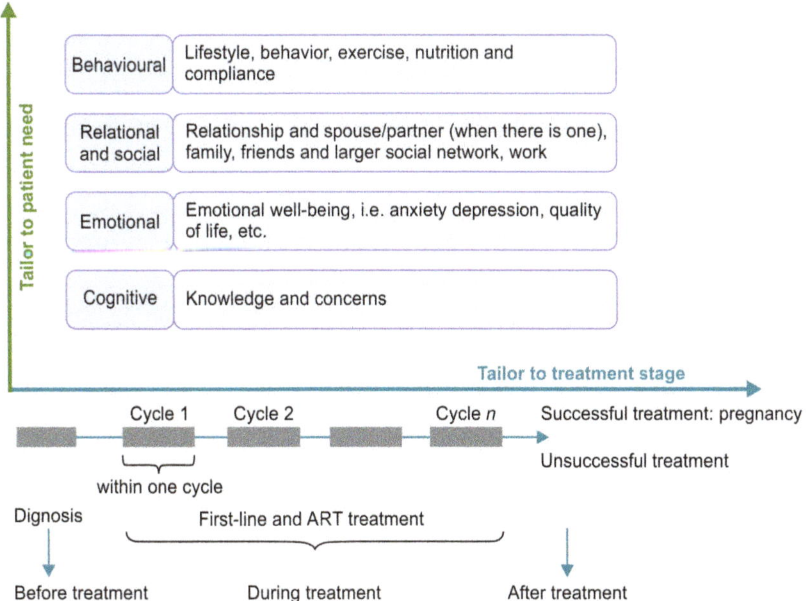

Fig. 1: Schematic representation of the guideline approach for the provision of psychosocial care tailored to specific infertility and assisted reproductive technology (ART) treatment stages and patient needs.
Adapted from: ESHRE 2015.

5. *Role of thromboprophylaxis:* It has been proposed that low molecular weight heparins (LMWH) have a possible role in successful implantation of the developing embryo through modulating a wide variety of proteins involved. It has been suggested that heparins can improve the apposition of the blastocyst and interfere with the apoptosis occurring during the implantation stage of a pregnancy. Two systematic reviews found that the administration of LMWH may increase clinical pregnancy and live birth rates in women undergoing IVF or intra cell sperm injection (ICSI). However, women undergoing ART who develop severe ovarian hyperstimulation syndrome, the ASH guideline panel *suggest* prophylactic antithrombotic therapy to prevent VTE.[5]

■ REFERENCES

1. Pinborg A, Loft A, AarisHenningsen AK, Rasmussen S, Andersen AN. Infant outcome of 957 singletons born after frozen embryo replacement: the Danish National Cohort Study 1995–2006. Fertil Steril. 2010;94:1320-7.
2. Jackson RA, Gibson KA, Wu YW, Croughan MS. Perinatal outcomes in singletons following in vitro fertilization: a meta-analysis. Obstet Gynecol. 2004;103:551-63.
3. Shevell T, Malone FD, Vidaver J, Porter TF, Luthy DA, Comstock CH, et al. Assisted reproductive technology and pregnancy outcome. Obstet Gynecol. 2005;106:1039-45.
4. Sinkey RG, Odibo AO, Dashe JS. Diagnosis and management of vasa previa. Society for Maternal–Fetal Medicine Consult Series #37. Am J Obstet Gynecol. 2015;213:615.
5. Bates SM, Rajasekhar A, Middeldorp S, McLintock C, Rodger MA, James AH, Vazquez SR, Greer IA, Riva JJ, Bhatt M, Schwab N. American Society of Hematology 2018 guidelines for management of venous thromboembolism: venous thromboembolism in the context of pregnancy. Blood advances. 2018;2(22):3317-59.

Assisted Reproductive Technology (Regulation) Act, 2021 and ART (Regulation) Rules, 2022: Is it Relevant for General Gynecologists?

Geetendra Sharma, SM Rahman

■ INTRODUCTION

Assisted Reproductive Technology (Regulation) Act 2021 and ART (Regulation) rules 2022 was passed by Indian Parliament to bring ART practice in India within the framework of law. Different provisions of ART (Regulation) Act and rules under have been debated by most of the ART clinicians and embryologists. Some modifications and clarifications of the bill have been brought by GOI.

■ IS IT RELEVANT FOR GENERAL GYNECOLOGISTS?

Yes, Ignorance of law is no excuse. It's important for general gynecologists to know the basic framework and provisions of the bill. Mostly because, a significant number of infertility patients are seen by general gynecologists (both in Government and Private setups). Initial workup is done by general gynecologists. Ovulation induction medications are prescribed by them and even IUI are performed by them sometimes. Then they prefer to refer patients to ART clinics when IVF is necessary.

■ BASIC PROVISIONS OF THE BILL, WHICH ARE IMPORTANT FOR EVERYONE

Level 1 Clinic (Registration Fees 50,000 INR for 5 Years)

Minimum staff: 1 Gynecologist (Qualification: The gynecologist shall be a medical post-graduate in gynecology and obstetrics).

Equipment and infrastructures: (i) Microscope, (ii) Centrifuge, (iii) Refrigerator (These are minimum requirement to get Registered).

No mention about size/shape/orientation of sterile and Non sterile zone.

Dos: Can perform OPD, Folliculometry by USG, Semen Preparation and IUI (including Donor IUI, hence, Donor Semen can be procured from any Registered ART Bank).

Cryopreservation facility: Fertility preservation of gametes can be done any malignancy treatment or Procedure.

Don'ts: Cannot perform Donor Gamete Cryopreservation or any ART Bank related work, IVF, ICSI, ET, PGT, Surrogacy and Research are prohibited.

Level 2 (Registration Fees: 2,00,000 INR for 5 Years)

Minimum staff: 1 Gynecologist, 1 Anesthetist, 1 embryologist and 1 Counselor. The additional staff at the level of Director and Andrologist may be employed but not mandatory.

Qualification:
Gynecologist: PG in OG with at least 50 OPU along with 3 years' experience in Infertility or MD or FNB with at least 3 years' experience.

Anesthetist: Anesthetist will be a medical post-graduate in Anesthesia.

Embryologist: Full time MCE with 3 years human ART laboratory experiences in handling human gametes and embryos; Full Time PhD (Thesis related to Clinical Embryology or ART or fertility) with additional one year of human ART laboratory experience in handling human gametes and embryos; MBBS or BVSc should have MCE (full time) with 2 years ART laboratory experience in handling human gametes and embryos; MSc in Biotech or Life Sciences minimum of one year of on-site, fulltime clinical embryology certified training in addition to 4 years' experience in handling human gametes and embryos in a registered ART level 2 clinic.

Counsellor: A person who is a graduate in Psychology or Clinical Psychology or Nursing or Life Sciences. Director: The director shall have a post-graduate degree in Medical or Life Sciences or Management Sciences.

Andrologist: The Andrologist in a clinic or a bank will be an MCh or DNB in Urology with special training in Diagnosing and Treating Male infertility.

For one time measure please refer to ART Regulation Rule Book 2022 Schedule 1, Part 1, A.c.

Equipment and Infrastructures

(a) Microscope; (b) Incubator (minimum 02 in number); (c) Laminar Airflow; (d) Sperm counting chambers; (e) Centrifuge; (f) Refrigerator; (g) Equipment for cryopreservation; (h) Ovum Aspiration Pump; (i) USG machine with transvaginal probe and needle guard; (j) Test tube warmer, and (k) Anesthesia resuscitation trolley. (These are minimum requirement to get Registered)

No mention about size/shape/physical requirement/orientation of sterile and non-sterile zone.

Dos: Can perform OPD, Folliculometry by USG, IUI, IVF, ICSI, PGT, Any Surgical Sperm Extraction Procedure i.e., TESA, PESA, TESE. They can perform any ART procedure including Donor IUI/IVF. Hence, donor sperm mandatorily is procured from any Registered ART Bank . They either can procure Donor Oocytes from any Registered ART Bank or preferably can perform Donor Oocyte retrieval, post Controlled ovarian Stimulation (as per ART Rule 2022, Section 13, sub section 1, clause c), and up to 7 Oocytes can be retrieved (as per ART Act 2021, Section 27, sub-Section 4). Those 7 Oocytes either be used for IVF/ICSI with Husband's Sperm of prespecified intending couple or can be fertilized with Donor Sperm if clinically intended (in case of aspermia, azoospermia or any poor sperm quality) or those 7 Oocytes may be frozen for future use for that intending couple only. Single Mother can go for IVF/ICSI with Donor Sperm if she is clinically indicated to avail IVF. Cryopreservation Facility: Donor Oocyte Freezing, Husband Sperm Freezing for back up, Wife's Oocytes Freezing for back up, 'Social' Egg or Sperm Freezing can be done for future self-use, Minor's or Adult's Sperm/Oocytes/ Testicular / Ovarian tissue Freezing can be done before any Malignancy treatment or Procedure and can be used for self-ART Cycle, in future post recovery from the disease, as per patient's wish.

SOME OTHER IMPORTANT POINTS FOR ALL GYNECOLOGIST TO KNOW

Q. Who can avail ART?

21–50 Years (female) 21–55 Years (male)

Q. Who can become Sperm Donor?

21–55 Years

Q. Who can become Oocyte Donor?

23–35 Years
Once in a life time
Non-compensated

Q. Who can avail surrogacy?

Patient/intending couple: 23–50 Years (female) 26–55 Years (male) (provided the intending couple have not had any surviving child biologically or through adoption or through surrogacy earlier).

Q. Who can become surrogate mother?

25–35 Years (female)
Once in a life time
Altruistic only.

Q. What are the single mother's age criteria to avail ART?
21–50 Years IUI/IVF (Normal as others)

Q. Can single mother can do IUI treatment?

Single mother can avail IUI treatment with Donor Sperm.

Q. Can OCI or PIO avail surrogacy in India?

Yes! Person of Indian origin can avail surrogacy in India.

Q. Can OCI or PIO avail ART or Donor ART in India?

Yes

 Q. Can foreigners avail ART service in India?

Yes

Q. Can foreigners avail donor cycle ART in India?

Yes

Q. Can foreigners avail surrogacy in India?

No. Only Person of Indian Origin with the permission of Appropriate Authority can avail Surrogacy in India.

Q. Can we perform PGT-A to check Embryo aneuploidy?

Yes, if the Patient has any "known, pre-existing heritable or genetic diseases", then according to the Act, PGT can be opted. This Medical Indication like previous history of Down syndrome with secondary infertility, failure history of IVF or RIF (Repeated Implantation Failure) or Unexplained infertility or Diminishing Ovarian Reserve or Higher Age Group, where chance of occurrence of aneuploidy is higher, those patients can opt for PGT-A.

Q. Does a gynecologist need to get registered under ART Regulation Act to practice Ovarian Stimulation (Up to HCG Trigger)/Ovulation Induction or Folliculometry?

For Folliculometry and Ovulation Induction with timed intercourse, no need get registered under this ART Act.

For Ovarian Stimulation, the gynecologist needs to be registered through the corresponding Level 2 ART Clinic where he is going to do the Oocyte retrieval, because Ovarian Stimulation and triggering is a part of an IVF Treatment.

Q. Can a Pathology center or any non-ART Center perform Semen Analysis?

Yes

Q. Can a Pathology center or any non-ART Center prepare Semen?

No

Q. Is Gamete Donation an Altruistic is Nature?

Yes, No Commercialization of Gamete Donation. But nowhere in Act or Rule it is mentioned that Gamete Donation is Altruistic in nature. Recent RTI Reply (DOHRE/R/E/22/00314, 11th Nov, 2022) confirms that any commercial gain is prohibited under this Act other than insurance coverage for a period of twelve months will be purchased by the commissioning couple or woman in favor of the oocyte donor.

Q. Is surrogacy an altruistic is nature?

Yes, truly Altruistic in nature. Commercial Surrogacy is strictly prohibited by Surrogacy Law. Surrogacy Regulation Act 2021, Section 2, Clause (b) is defining clearly that "altruistic surrogacy" means the surrogacy in which no charges, expenses, fees, remuneration or monetary incentive of whatever nature, except the medical expenses and such other prescribed expenses incurred on surrogate mother and the insurance coverage for the surrogate mother, are given to the surrogate mother or her dependents or her representative; Though the definition of "Insurance" is common in ART and Surrogacy Regulation Act both, but the above mentioned Clause (b) entirely prohibits any kind of monitory transaction like daily wages or transportation expenses whatsoever., other than only Medical or related expenses on actuals.

Q. Insurance coverage for how many years for oocyte donor and surrogate mother?

One year for oocyte donor and 36 months for surrogate mother.

Q. Within how many days, ART Bank has to upload all information to the national database?

One month from the date of receipt of such information.

Q. Who can come and search the premises of ART Clinic/Bank or Surrogacy Clinic?

If the National Board, the National Registry, the State Board or Appropriate Authority has reason to believe that an offense under this Act has been or is being committed at any facility using assisted reproductive technology, such Board or any officer authorized in this behalf may, subject to such rules as may be prescribed, enter and search at all reasonable times with such assistance, if any, as such Board or officer considers necessary, such facility using assisted reproductive technology and examine any record, register, document, book, pamphlet, advertisement or any other material object found therein and seize the same, if the said Board has reason to believe that it may furnish evidence of the commission of an offense punishable under this Act.

Q. Online National Registry of ART and Surrogacy?

www.registry.artsurrogacy.gov.in

Q. Any government official website related to ART and surrogacy?

www.artsurrogacy.gov.in

Q. From which date all consents and Papers to be kept according to the New ART and Surrogacy Act and Rule?

As and when Act and Rule came into effect—from 25th January 2022 onwards (Whatever mentioned in the ART and Surrogacy Regulation Act 2021) Post 7th June 2022 onwards (Whatever mentioned in the ART Rule 2022) Post 21st June 2022 onwards (Whatever mentioned in the Surrogacy Rule 2022).

The Legal Road to Surrogacy: Who, What, When, and Where

Chaitali Datta Ray

■ INTRODUCTION

The Surrogacy (Regulation) Act, 2021 received the assent of the President of India on 25th of December, 2021 and brought about a paradigm procedural shift in the practice of Surrogacy in India.

■ BOARD AND APPROPRIATE AUTHORITY[1]

The Act led to the constitution of National Assisted Reproductive Technology and Surrogacy Board, State Assisted Reproductive Technology and Surrogacy Boards and appointment of appropriate authorities for regulation and monitoring of the practice and process of surrogacy.

The radical conversion of surrogacy from commercial to solely altruistic, along with the inclusion of various mandatory certificates prior to the actual clinical process, has led to a great a deal of confusion among the couples applying for Surrogacy, along with the medical professionals attempting to relieve them of their suffering.

■ RELEVANT TERMINOLOGY DEFINED IN THE ACT[2]

Surrogacy: A practice whereby one woman bears and gives birth to a child for an intending couple with the intention of handing over such child to the intending couple after the birth.

Gestational surrogacy: A practice whereby a surrogate mother carries a child for the intending couple through implantation of embryo in her womb and the child is not genetically related to the surrogate mother.

Intending couple: This refers to a couple with a medical indication necessitating gestational surrogacy and who intend to become parents through surrogacy.

Intending woman: This refers to a woman who is a widow or divorcee, who intends to avail of surrogacy.

Surrogate mother: A woman who agrees to bear a child (who is genetically related to the intending couple or intending woman) through surrogacy, from the implantation of embryo in her womb.

STEPWISE PROCEDURE TO BE FOLLOWED BY THE INTENDING COUPLE/INTENDING WOMAN

First step
↓

The Intending couple or intending woman must first apply to CMOH office of their respective district for issue of:

CERTIFICATE OF MEDICAL INDICATION (FROM DISTRICT MEDICAL BOARD)[3]

District medical board: It means a medical board under the Chairpersonship of Chief Medical Officer or Chief Civil Surgeon or Joint Director of Health Services of the district and comprising of at least two other specialists, namely, the chief gynecologist or obstetrician and chief pediatrician of the district.

Medical Indications Necessitating Gestational Surrogacy[4]

A woman may opt for surrogacy if:

a. She has no uterus or has a missing or abnormal uterus (like hypoplastic uterus or intrauterine adhesions or thin endometrium or small unicornuate uterus, T-shaped uterus) or if the uterus is surgically removed due to any medical conditions such as gynecological cancer.

b. Intended parent or woman has repeatedly failed to conceive after multiple In vitro fertilization or Intracytoplasmic sperm injection attempts (Recurrent implantation failure).

c. Intended parent or woman has multiple pregnancy losses resulting from an unexplained medical reason or unexplained graft rejection due to exaggerated immune response.

d. Intended parent or woman has any illness that makes it impossible for a woman to carry a pregnancy to viability or pregnancy that is life threatening.

↓

Simultaneously they must also obtain:

Order Concerning the Parentage and Custody of the Child to be Born Through Surrogacy[5]

This must be passed by a court of the Magistrate of the first class or above on an application made by the intending couple or the intending woman and the surrogate mother, which shall be the birth affidavit after the surrogate child is born.

Affidavit of Insurance Coverage[6]

This must be of such amount and in such manner as may be prescribed in favor of the surrogate mother for a period of thirty-six months covering postpartum delivery complications. It must be from an insurance company or an agent recognized by the Insurance Regulatory and Development Authority.

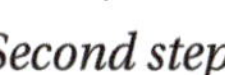

Second step
They must appear before state appropriate authority for issue of:

Certificate of Essentiality[7]

For issuance of this they/she must bring the following documents:
- Certificate of Medical Indication
- Order concerning the Parentage and Custody of the Child
- Affidavit on insurance coverage.

Certificate of Elligibility[8]

There are certain criteria to be fulfilled for the Intending Couple/Woman to be eligible for Surrogacy as per the Act.

Criteria to be fulfilled by the intending couple:
- They must be of Indian origin.
- The intending couple is married.
- They are between the ages of 23 to 50 years in case of female and between 26 to 55 years in case of male on the day of certification.
- The intending couple have not had any surviving child biologically or through adoption or through surrogacy earlier.

Exception: The intending couple has a child who is mentally or physically challenged or suffers from life threatening disorder or fatal illness with no permanent cure. This is approved by the appropriate authority with due medical certificate from a District Medical Board.

Criteria to be fulfilled by the intending woman:
- She must be of Indian origin.
- She must be a widow or divorcee.
- She must be between the ages of 35 to 45 years.
  Other criteria are similar to that of intending couple.

In this respect they must bring the following documents:
- Aadhaar card
- Proof of marriage/marriage certificate (If applicable)/divorce certificate (if applicable) or other relevant documents pertaining to this criteria
- Proof of age/birth certificate/10th certificate/or any equivalent
- Proof that they do not have any surviving child biologically or through adoption or through surrogacy earlier.

↓

Simultaneously the intending couple/woman shall approach the
appropriate authority with a willing woman
who agrees to act as a surrogate mother

Surrogate mothers must apply to state appropriate authority for eligibility
certficate[11]

Criteria to be fulfilled by the surrogate mother:
- She must be an ever married woman.
- She must be having a child of her own.
- She must be between the ages of 25 to 35 years on the day of implantation.
- She must possess a certificate of medical and psychological fitness for surrogacy and surrogacy procedures from a registered medical practitioner.

She must bring:
- Aadhaar
- Proof of marriage/Marriage Certificate (If applicable)
- Proof of age/Birth certificate/10th certificate/or any equivalent
- Proof of at least one living child
- Affidavit that she has not been a surrogate mother before
- Certificate of medical and psychological fitness for surrogacy and surrogacy procedures from a registered medical practitioner
- Consent certificate as per FORM 2 of as per surrogacy (Regulation) Rules, 2022

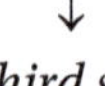

Third step
With above documents they must apply to National Board for:
Certificate of recommendation[9,10] in form 1 of surrogacy (Regulation)
rules, 2022

Fourth step
With certificate of recommendation they may approach a registered
surrogacy clinic for initiation of the surrogacy procedure

The director/in-charge of the surrogacy clinic and person qualified to do so:
Must be satisfied (recorded in writing) that the following conditions have been fulfilled:
1. Certificate of medical indication from a district medical board
2. Order concerning the parentage and custody of the child to be born through surrogacy[5]
3. Affidavit of insurance coverage[6] for the surrogate mother
4. Eligibility certificateof the surrogate mother issued by appropriate authority
5. Consent certificate of the surrogate mother.

■ SOME IMPORTANT CONTACT DETAILS

- The National ART and Surrogacy Board: Chairperson, National ART and Surrogacy Board, 2nd Floor, IRCS Building 1, Red Cross Road, New Delhi-110001 Email: sn.jasra38@nic.in
- **State appropriate authority:* Chairperson or State Nodal Officer, State Appropriate Authority under ART and Surrogacy Act
- ***District medical board:* Chief Medical Officer of Health and Chairperson of Dist. Med Board.

■ FURTHER READING

1. The Surrogacy (Regulation) Act, 2021, Chapter 5.
2. The Surrogacy (Regulation) Act, 2021, Chapter I, 2. (1).
3. Surrogacy (Regulation) Act, 2021, Chapter III Regulation of Surrogacy and Surrogacy Procedures.
4. As per Surrogacy (Regulation) Rules, 2022: Rule 14.
5. Surrogacy (Regulation) Act, 2021, Chapter III Regulation of Surrogacy and Surrogacy Procedures, 4 (iii) (a)(II).
6. Chapter III Regulation of Surrogacy and Surrogacy Procedures, 4 (iii) (a)(III)).
7. As per Chapter III Regulation of Surrogacy and Surrogacy Procedures 4 (iii)(a).
8. As per Chapter III Regulation of Surrogacy and Surrogacy Procedures 4 (iii)(b).
9. The Surrogacy (Regulation) Act, 2021,Chapter I Preliminary: 2 (1) (e).
10. Chapter III Regulation of Surrogacy and Surrogacy Procedures: 4 (ii) (a); section 17.
11. Surrogacy (Regulation) Act, 2021, Chapter III, 4 (iii) (b); Regulation of Surrogacy and Surrogacy Procedures.